WRITTEN LANGUAGE DISORDERS

NEUROPSYCHOLOGY AND COGNITION

VOLUME 2

The purpose of the Neuropsychology and Cognition series is to bring out volumes that promote understanding in topics relating brain and behavior. It is intended for use by both clinicians and research scientists in the fields of neuropsychology, cognitive psychology, psycholinguistics, speech and hearing, as well as education. Examples of topics to be covered in the series would relate to memory, language acquisition and breakdown, reading, attention, developing and aging brain. By addressing the theoretical, empirical, and applied aspects of brain-behavior relationships, this series will try to present the information in the fields of neuropsychology and cognition in a coherent manner.

The titles published in this series are listed at the end of this volume.

WRITTEN LANGUAGE DISORDERS

Edited by

R. MALATESHA JOSHI

Oklahoma State University

KLUWER ACADEMIC PUBLISHERS

DORDRECHT / BOSTON / LONDON

Library of Congress Cataloging-in-Publication Data

Written language disorders / edited by R. Malatesha Joshi.
          p.   cm. -- (Neuropsychology and cognition ; 2)
    Includes bibliographical references and index.
    ISBN 0-7923-0902-2 (U.S. : acid-free paper)
    1. Agraphia. 2. Alexia.   I. Joshi, R. Malatesha.   II. Series.
    RC429.W75 1991
    616.85'53--dc20   90-44392

ISBN 0-7923-0902-2

Published by Kluwer Academic Publishers,
P.O. Box 17, 3300 AA Dordrecht, The Netherlands.

Kluwer Academic Publishers incorporates the publishing programmes of
D. Reidel, Martinus Nijhoff, Dr W. Junk and MTP Press.

Sold and distributed in the U.S.A. and Canada
by Kluwer Academic Publishers,
101 Philip Drive, Norwell, MA 02061, U.S.A.

In all other countries, sold and distributed
by Kluwer Academic Publishers Group.
P.O. Box 322, 3300 AH Dordrecht, The Netherlands.

Printed on acid-free paper

Printed in the Netherlands

TABLE OF CONTENTS

PREFACE

Although anecdotal reports of loss of once-acquired reading ability was noticed in the individuals who had sustained brain damage as early as the year A.D. 30, systematic enquires of alexia were not undertaken until the latter part of the nineteenth century. The two anatomo-pathological studies carried out by Dejerine in 1891 and 1892 mark the beginning of scholarly investigation of reading failure. Interestingly, the study of developmental reading disability also began to receive attention at about the same time when Pringle Morgan described the case of a 14-year-old boy who had great difficulty in reading and writing. Since then sporadic reports of developmental reading-writing failure began to appear in medical and educational journals even though such investigation went on at an unhurried pace. In the past two decades, however, the situation has changed enormously and hundreds of articles that have investigated developmental and acquired cognitive disabilities have been published. Disorders of spoken language and written language are two areas that have been extensively addressed by these articles. Those who study disorders of language come from a wide variety of backgrounds and their reports are also published in a variety of journals. The purpose of the present volume is to bring some important research findings of written language disorders together and present them in a coherent format.

In Chapter 1, Joshi and Aaron challenge the validity of the notion of the putative "poor speller but good reader'. They contend that even though superficially some poor spellers may appear to be good readers, thorough investigation of these subjects would reveal subtle reading disabilities. They support this conclusion with evidence collected from three college students.

In Chapter 2, Maul and Ehri describe experiments that tested the hypothesis that normal spellers use the same processes to read and spell whereas poor spellers use different processes to read and spell. Based on the results of their investigation, they conclude that both good and poor spellers use phonological as well as visual-orthographic processes to spell and read.

One of the often quoted reasons for the high incidence of reading and spelling problems in the English language is that there is no consistent relationship between the written and spoken forms of English words. However, investigations that have addressed this issue from a morphophonemic perspective have concluded that, to a large extent, English language is a rule-governed system of communication. The influence of morphophonological knowledge on the writing performance of very young children is examined by Rubin. The results of this study are presented in Chapter 3.

Whether or not brain damage has differential effect on linguistic and perceptual process is examined in Chapter 4 by Caramazza and Hillis. Their investigations of neuropsychological patients reveal that cognitive skills such as reading and spelling are dissociable. In Chapter 5, Miceli presents a model of the spelling processes based on the evidence collected from patients whose cognitive skills are impaired. This model can accommodate the individual differences that are seen in the performance of these subjects.

In the next chapter, Lebrun and De Vreese examine the different forms of alexias. They conclude that there is a great deal of variability among different individuals as far as the nature of symptoms and the rate of recovery are concerned. These authors conclude that because of such variability, a unitary theory of alexia may not be possible.

In Chapter 7, Lebrun, Devreaux, and Leleux describe the seldom investigated graphomotor disability called "Writer's cramp". The authors point out that there is no uniformity of symptoms in writer's cramp and conclude the chapter with recommendations for diagnosis and therapy.

In contrast to dyslexia, the reading disability known as hyperlexia has a rather brief history. The syndrome of hyperlexia includes superior word-decoding skill and an associated poor comprehension. Rispens and van Berckelaer describe the syndrome in Chapter 8 and present criteria for the diagnosis of hyperlexia.

In Chapter 9, Luelsdorff and Eyland propose a psycholinguistic model derived from observations made on the spelling performance of bilinguals. Because bilingual subjects who become alexic are rare, the study of bilinguals provides a new perspective for the investigation of the neuro-psychology of language processing.

In spite of the fact that the articles presented in this book address varying aspects of the written language, they present a single theme, namely the understanding of the neuropsychology of written language processing. Authors of the chapters contained in this volume are well known for their research in this area and I thank them for their contributions.

R. MALATESHA JOSHI

LIST OF CONTRIBUTORS

P. G. AARON, Department of Educational Psychology, Indiana State University, Terre Haute, Indiana, 47809, U.S.A.

ALFONSO CARAMAZZA, Cognitive Science Center, The Johns Hopkins University, Baltimore, Maryland, 21218, U.S.A.

FRANCOISE DEVREUX, Neurolinguistics Department, School of Medicine, Vrije Universiteit Brussel, 1090 Brussels, Belgium.

LUC DE VREESE, Neurolinguistics Department, School of Medicine, Vrije Universiteit Brussel, 1090 Brussels, Belgium.

LINNEA C. EHRI, Division of Education, College of Letters and Sciences, University of California, Davis, California, 95616, U.S.A.

E. ANN EYLAND, Macquaire University, North Ryde, NSW 2109, Australia.

ARGYE E. HILLIS, Cognitive Science Center, The Johns Hopkins University, Baltimore, Maryland, 21218, U.S.A.

R. MALATESHA JOSHI, Department of Curriculum and Instruction, Oklahoma State University, Stillwater, Oklahoma 74078, U.S.A.

YVAN LEBRUN, Neurolinguistics Department, School of Medicine, Vrije Universiteit Brussel, 1090 Brussels, Belgium.

CHANTAL LELEUX, Neurolinguistics Department, School of Medicine, Vrije Universiteit Brussel, 1090 Brussels, Belgium.

PHILIP A. LUELSDORFF, Universitat Regensburg, 8400 Regensburg, Federal Republic of Germany.

BEVERLY D. K. MAUL, West Davis Intermediate School, 1207 Sycamore Lane, Davis, CA 95616 U.S.A.

GABRIELE MICELI, Clinica Neurologica, Universita Cattolica, Largo A. Gemelli 8, 00168, Rome, Italy.

JAN RISPENS, Faculteit der Sociale Wetenschappen, Vakgroep Kinderstudies, Postbus 80.140, 3508 TC Utrecht, The Netherlands

HYLA RUBIN, Graduate Department of Speech Pathology, Faculty of Medicine, University of Toronto, Toronto, Canada M5G 1L4.

I. A. VAN BERCKELAER, Faculteit der Sociale Wetenschappen, University of Leiden, 2334 BP Leiden, The Netherlands.

R. MALATESHA JOSHI AND P. G. AARON

DEVELOPMENTAL READING AND SPELLING DISABILITIES: ARE THESE DISSOCIABLE?

1. INTRODUCTION

Studies of developmental dyslexia in children suggest that poor spelling is an inevitable concomitant of poor reading (Cook, 1981; Gerber, 1984; Nelson and Warrington, 1976). This should come as no surprise since it appears that spelling-sound relational rules are used in both reading and spelling (Baron *et al.*, 1980) and that many dyslexic subjects are deficient in these grapheme-phoneme conversion skills (Aaron, 1989; Aaron *et al.*, 1984; Perfetti and Hogaboam, 1975; Snowling, 1980). A recent study by Waters *et al.* (1985), which specifically examined the question whether children use similar processes to read and spell words, found that third grade children, regardless of their ability level, used spelling-sound corre-spondences in both reading and spelling. Conversely, studies of spelling ability also have shown that poor spellers are deficient in decoding skills (Spache, 1940) and that acquisition of spelling involves progressive inter-nalization of orthographic rules (Beers, 1980). These observations are further buttressed by the classical neurology doctrine that writing dis-orders do not exist in isolation but occur simultaneously and equally often with disorders of speech and the reason why this view has persisted so long is that it is supported by the bulk of clinical experience (Margolin, 1984).

Viewed in the light of these observations, the few published reports of the occurrence of pure developmental spelling disability without being accompanied by reading deficits present a paradox. Spelling disability that reportedly exists along with normal reading ability is referred to as "developmental spelling retardation" (Nelson and Warrington, 1974), "unexpected spelling problems" (Frith, 1980), "spelling only retardation" (Jorm, 1983), and "specific spelling problems" (Frith, 1984). Occasionally, a more descriptive lable such as "poor spellers who are good readers" (Frith, 1980, p. 514) is used.

The findings of a few recently published neuropsychological studies also suggest a possible dissociation between spelling and reading. One frequently quoted study is by Beauvois and Derouesne (1979) which proposed a dissociation between the phonological route to reading and the phonological route to spelling because the patient was impaired in reading but not in spelling (cf, Temple, 1985a). It should, however, be noted that R.G., the patient studied by Beauvois and Derouesne, committed some spelling mistakes and that "the patient's writing was not entirely normal"

R. M. Joshi (ed.), Written Language Disorders, 1—24.
© 1991 *Kluwer Academic Publishers. Printed in the Netherlands.*

(p. 1120). Other neuropsychological studies claim a dissociation between reading and spelling because the etiology and symptoms of the reading disorder are categorically different from those of the spelling disorder. For instance, Hatfield and Patterson (1983) describe a patient whose oral reading could be interpreted as that of a surface dyslexic but whose spelling was reminiscent of phonological dysgraphia. Temple (1985b) has described a developmental dyslexic who, according to her, was not a surface dyslexic but was a surface dysgraphic. These cases are more fully discussed at the end of this chapter and alternative interpretations are suggested.

The existence of some putative adults who are proficient readers but inconsistent spellers is also often cited as evidence of the independence of reading and spelling processes. Hatfield and Patterson (1983) address this "curious discrepancy" between reading and writing skills in normal and even highly literate adults and cite their professional colleague R.P. as an example.

A possible resolution to the controversy of whether or not spelling and reading are independent processes could be found in a statement by Bryant and Bradley (1980) that they have encountered children of 11 and 12 who read well but spell appallingly but who, later on at around the age of 13, experience serious reading difficulties because they are unable to use phonological strategy to meet the increased demands of reading. In view of this statement, adults who are poor spellers but who, nevertheless, appear to be proficient readers, probably manage to read well by using a whole word visual recognition strategy. If sufficiently well developed, such a strategy can mask the underlying phonological deficit. Such a strategy, however, will fail in spelling because, unlike reading, spelling a word is a recall task and the appropriate letter strings have to be generated on the basis of phonology. If it could be shown that skilled reading could be accomplished in spite of poor spelling ability, it would also demonstrate that the phonological route is not necessary for skilled reading. The implications of such a finding for models of reading are obvious. It will be argued in this paper that such a condition does not exist and that upon close scrutiny, the so-called "good reader but poor speller" does show reading deficiencies at least under some unusual conditions. In addition to these theoretical implications, the relationship between spelling and reading is of practical value for the reason that if spelling and reading are separable skills, recent developments in early reading instruction that approach reading through writing (Write to Read) are based on insecure foundations.

2. CASE STUDIES

Three college students who approached the psychology clinic seeking help to improve their spelling skills were used as subjects. All the three subjects reported that poor spelling was their persisting problems. They also said that they did not experience any reading difficulties and considered themselves to be good readers.

Case 1: S.H. S.H. is a 23-year-old left-handed male currently working towards a bachelor's degree in technology. He uses his left hand to write or cut with scissors and his right hand for sport activities such as throwing the baseball. His mother also had a similar pattern of mixed hand use. His childhood health history was uneventful, and medical examination before entering the army indicated no physical or sensory handicaps. S.H. reported that he was required to repeat Grades 1 and 5 because he was a slow reader. At present he considers himself to be a good reader but a poor speller.

Case 2:   P.C. P.C. is a 29-year-old right-handed female who is in the second year of college. She considers herself to have been an average student in elementary and high schools. After high school, her formal education had an erratic history with periods of work interspersed with school. P.C. could not recall her mother or siblings having had any reading difficulties; she could not provide any information about her father who left the family when she was quite young. P.C. has had a normal health history except for a bicycle accident which left her unconscious for a few minutes. During interviews, she was quite articulate even though somewhat impulsive.

Case 3: O.C. O.C. is a 31-year-old female who is currently working towards a Master's degree in Special Education. She is right-handed and reports that she had had no reading problems either before or during her college years. Her educational career was interrupted by a few years of service with a volunteer organization. She had had no serious health problems except for occasional migraine headaches. There is no family history of any serious reading disability. Like the other two subjects, O.C. considers herself a good reader but a poor speller.

Three college students who were normal readers served as members of a control group. The experimental and control subjects were administered the Wechsler's Adult Intelligence Scale and the Stanford Diagnostic Reading Test (Karlsen *et al.*, 1974). The Comprehension subtest of the Stanford Reading Test was administered without time restrictions. The results are shown in Table 1.

3. HYPOTHESIS

Five predictions were made in order to test the validity of the hypothesis

TABLE 1
WAIS-R and the Stanford Diagnostic Reading Test Results

| Subject | WAIS-IQ | | | Reading test* | | | |
	VIQ	PIQ	FIQ	Reading rate	Vocabulary	Decoding	Comprehension**
S.H.	110	116	113	5.5	12.2	9.0	13.0
P.C.	97	110	103	9.2	12.5	7.2	13.0
O.C.	96	96	96	5.9	13.0	13.0	13.0

 * Grade level
** Untimed subtest

that the "good reader but poor speller" does have subtle reading deficits. These predictions were generated on the basis of rationale derived from the following information.

Neuropsychological studies indicate that reading may involve the flexible use of two processes, a direct visual accessing of the lexicon and a phonological conversion operation. The reported cases of deep and phonological dyslexias (Beauvois and Dérouésne, 1979; Marshall and Newcombe, 1973) show that direct visual lexical accessing alone is insufficient to carry out *accurate* reading.

Similarly, it appears that accurate spelling involves a direct visual route and a phonemic-graphemic route (Nelson, 1980). Developmental studies of spelling and reading (Bissex, 1980; Bradley and Bryant, 1979; Chomsky, 1970; Read, 1971) suggest that pre-school children use a primitive phonological strategy for spelling and a whole-word strategy for reading. However, as noted earlier, when these children progress through school, shifts occur in their reading and spelling strategies (Bryant and Bradley, 1980; Gentry, 1982). Ultimately, they become fluent readers and good spellers by becoming adept in the flexible use of the direct visual and phonological strategies.

Studies by Calfee *et al.* (1969) and Venezky (1976) show that the phoneme-grapheme conversion rules used in spelling words are acquired in stages. Based on these studies, we devised a spelling test that was made up of words the spelling of which reflected increasingly complex grapheme-phoneme relational rules. The spelling test was then administered to a group of 70 children from Grades 2 through 6. Analysis of results showed that the phoneme-grapheme relational rules used in spelling are acquired progressively as children grow older (Table 2). For instance, the $c = /k/$ (as in "cake") was mastered by all second grade normal readers, whereas only 65.8% of these children knew the use of $c = /s/$ (as in "cent"). This difference cannot be attributed to word frequency effect since the word "cent" has a frequency higher than that of the word "cake".

TABLE 2
Percent of children from Grades 2 through 6 who produced correct spellings
(normal readers)

Rule	Target words (high frequency)	Percent correct	Target words (low frequency)	Percent correct	Mean percent correct
1. Initial c ?/k/	cat, cold	100	cake, cape	100	100.0
2. Initial g → /g/	girl, game	99	gift, gum	99	99.0
3. Terminal g → /g/	dog, sing	100	flag, hung	91	95.5
4. Middle g → /g/	begin, eggs	93	hanging, forget	98	95.5
5. Terminal g → /dʒ/	page, edge	88.2	merge, ledge	92	89.8
6. Middle g → /dʒ/	larger, region	83	digit, rigid	83.7	86.5
7. Initial ch → /tʃ/	children, chance	76.7	chess, chap	90	83.5
8. Initial g ?/dʒ/	gentle, giant	73.4	germ, gender	50	61.7
9. Middle c → /k/	uncle, fact	59	local, picnic	88	66.6
10. Initial c → /s/	city, certain	59	cent, circus	77	65.8
11. Rule of e	care, bite	52	spare, cute	48	50.0
12. Middle c → /s/	except, faces	40.7	concern, council	27.7	34.2
13. Compound vowels	daughter, aunt	31.5	build, couch	26	28.8

Words that contained vowel digraphs (e.g., "au" and "ou") were the most difficult ones to spell correctly.

On the basis of these observations, it is suspected that the "spelling only retarded" subjects are able to acquire the elementary grapheme-phoneme relational rules but fail to make progress beyond these initial stages. For this reason, even though their spelling errors would appear to be phonology based, the misspellings of the "poor speller but good reader" are, indeed, the result of the use of elementary sound-to-spelling relational rules and a failure to use the appropriate but more complex rules. For example, misspellings such as *city* → "sity" and *haul* → "hale" committed by them indicate a failure to use the c → /s/ rule and the digraph *au* rather than the mastery of the phonological rules. From this perspective, the so-called phonological spellings are really products of arrested phonological skill. By adopting a whole-word reading strategy, the "spelling only retarded" subject can, however, avoid the use of higher order GPC rules and accomplish certain amount of reading comprehension. Such a subject, however, will encounter difficulties in reading pronunciable nonwords as well as connected prose which contains unfamiliar and low-frequency words that require phonologic decoding. The extra effort spent in decoding unfamiliar and low-frequency words will also make the subject a relatively slow reader. Since the whole-word strategy obviates phonological rules, reading performance of regular and irregular words of these subjects is not likely to be different from each other. Spelling, being a recall task, is more affected by the phonological conversion deficiency than reading is.

Experimental studies show that there is a noticeable difference in the retrieval of words belonging to the open- and closed-class vocabularies (Bradley *et al.*, 1980; Kean, 1977). It is also known that children with reading disabilities find it more difficult to learn to read function words correctly than content words (Bruskin and Blank, 1984; Jolly, 1981). A diminished ability to recall function words has also been observed in tachistoscopic studies of adolescent dyslexics (Aaron *et al.*, 1985). Even though the mechanisms used in the processing of function words may not be the same as the ones used in the reading of pseudowords (Funnell, 1983), a difference in the processing of words belonging to the open and closed classes of words has been observed in some cases of acquired dyslexia (Marshall and Newcombe, 1973; Marshall, 1984). Thus, it is reasonable to expect the reading of function words (and inflexional morphemes) by the "spelling only retarded" subject to be different from his reading of content words.

For the above-stated reasons, the individual who has pure spelling disability is expected also to show signs of specific reading disability. The validity of this hypothesis was evaluated by generating the following five predictions and then testing them.

1. Because of a dependency on the visual-direct access strategy in reading, the "spelling only retarded" subjects will correctly read more high-frequency words than low-frequency words. Thus, word frequency and familiarity will have effects that exceed those seen in reading by normal readers.
2. Not being proficient in the use of grapheme-phoneme conversion rules, these subjects will commit many errors in reading pronunciable non-words.
3. Not being facile in the use of phonological conversion strategies, these subjects will be slow readers; in addition, their oral reading will contain an unsually large number of errors.
4. Since these subjects depend on a direct visual semantic lexical-access strategy for reading, their performance will not differ in the reading of regular and irregular words.
5. Their capacity to process function words and inflected suffixes would be relatively poor as compared to that of content words.

4. PROCEDURES AND FINDINGS

TASK 1: *Reading and spelling of low- and high-frequency words.* A list of 75 low-frequency words and another list of 75 high-frequency words (Carroll *et al.*, 1971) were prepared. An effort was made to match the words in the two lists for number of syllables (see Appendix). All the words in List 1 fell approximately above a frequency of 90 and those in

List 2 fell below 90 per 5,088,721 words of running text. Another important factor that governed the selection of these words was developmental spelling-pronunciation rules collected from different published reports (Dewey, 1970; Venezky, 1970, 1976; Wijk, 1966) as well as from our own study presented in Table 2. The words in the list thus reflect increasing complexity of spelling-pronunciation rules and are intended to test the subjects' ability to generate the appropriate pronunciation when certain morphophonemes occur in the initial, medial, and final positions.

These words were presented, one at a time, for a period of 500 milliseconds per word on an Apple II minicomputer monitor. The inter-stimulus interval was controlled by the subjects. The oral responses of the subjects were recorded. A week after the reading task was administered, the subjects were asked to spell these words by writing to dictation. Each word was first read by the experimenter, was followed by a sentence in which it was embedded, and was read once again.

Result. The numbers of words misread and misspelled by the subjects are shown in Table 3 and in Appendix. P.C. read all the 75 high-frequency words correctly, whereas S.H. and O.C. misread one word each. In contrast, S.H., P.C., and O.C. misread 3, 5, and 11 low-frequency words respectively. The misreadings were almost always due to the substitution of visually similar but higher frequency words (e.g., *benign* → "begin", *genus* → "genius"; *garnet* → "garment": *porridge* → "partridge"). These results show that word frequency has an effect on the reading performance of these subjects. An effect of this magnitude was not seen in the reading of the control subjects.

TABLE 3
Number of low- and high-frequency words misread and misspelled*

Frequency	S.H. Reading	S.H. Spelling	P.C. Reading	P.C. Spelling	O.C. Reading	O.C. Spelling	Controls ($n = 3$) Reading	Controls ($n = 3$) Spelling
High	1	15	0	10	1	9	0.0	0.0
Low	3	27	5	20	11	22	1.6	2.0

* There are 75 words in each category.

The three subjects committed many more spelling errors than reading errors. Here too, word-frequency effect could be observd. When these errors were analyzed on the basis of spelling to pronunciation rules, it was seen that, while certain high-frequency words were spelled correctly, low-frequency words based on the same rules were misspelled. Examples of words of differing frequencies but based on the same spelling-pronunciation rules that were spelled correctly and incorrectly are shown in Table 4.

Examples from Table 4 show that the subject were unable to apply the proper rules in spelling unfamiliar words even though they spelled correctly familiar words based on the same rules. These observations lead to the conclusion that the subjects have not mastered the rules of spelling but depend on some other strategy, possibly rote visual memory, to spell words. When such a strategy is not available (as in the case of words they are not familiar with), they are forced to use the elementary phoneme-grapheme relational rules they possess. The application of an inappropriate elementary rule in the place of a complex rule inevitably leads to spelling errors even though such errors create an impression of a dependence on phonology for spelling.

TABLE 4
A sample of words spelled correctly and incorroectly by the three subjects

Spelling rule	Word spelled correctly	Word spelled incorrectly
$c \rightarrow /s/$	*cent* (364)*; *central* (287)	*cede* (3) "sede"; *censor* (2) "sensor"
final *e*	*cheese* (236); *cake* (244); *gate* (267)	*chrome* (13) "chrome"; *gentle* (200) "gentl", "gentel"; *gale* (27) "gail", "gal"; *eclipse* (31) "eclips"
$ch \rightarrow /k/$	*chemical* (376); *character* (242)	*charisma* (2) "crisma"
$gi, ge \rightarrow /dʒ/$	*religion* (179); caged (240)	*rigid* (49) "ridget", "ridgible"; *legible* (10) "ledgeble"
silent *g*	*sign* (615)	*resign* (16) "resin"; *foreign* (263) "forgin"; *benign* (6) "benine"
secondary vowel *au*	*aunt* (390); *author* (219)	*haul* (53) "hale"
$che \rightarrow /tʃ/$	*pitcher* (114)	*bachelor* (9) "bachlor"; *luncheon* (31) "lunch on"

* Figures in parenthesis refer to word frequency

TASK 2: *Reading and spelling of nonwords.* Two different procedures were used to assess the subjects' ability to read pronunciable nonwords. The first procedure utilized a list of 50 nonwords that was constructed on the basis of the spelling-pronunciation rules that were used to create high- and low-frequency word lists described above (see Appendix). The nonwords differed from real words in one or two letters. For example, knowledge of the pronunciation rule $c \rightarrow /s/$ was tested by the words "cept", "recide", and "bace". Each word was presented on the minicomputer monitor as was in Task 1 and the subjects' responses were taped.

More than a month later, the same list of nonwords was administered as a spelling test. The subjects were forewarned that they were going to hear nonwords and that no such words exist. They were required to repeat the nonword before writing it.

The second procedure used a Gerbrands projection tachistoscope with a rear-view screen. Eighty 3-letter nouns, 80 function words, 80 pronunciable nonwords (CVC), an 80 nonpronunciable trigrams (CCC) were typed on cards and made into slides. Each slide had four stimuli of the same category arranged one below the other. There were 20 slides in each of the four categories of stimuli. After alerting a subject, each slide was presented for a duration of 500 milliseconds and as soon as the stimulus disappeared from the screen, the subject reported as many words as possible. One of the experimenters recorded the subject's responses. These word lists were not presented as a spelling task.

Result. The data obtained from these two procedures are shown in Table 5. The results obtained through the two different procedures show clearly that the subjects are very poor in reading nonwords. The reading errors are shown in the Appendix. The tendency to substitute real words for pseudowords (lexicalization) was observed both in reading and spelling. Of the 14, 11, and 20 words misread by S.H., P.C., and O.C., respectively, 10, 6, and 12 were lexicalizations. Examples of lexicalization common to all the three subjects were: *boncer* → "bouncer"; *ounch* → "ounce"; and *kot* → "coat".

Data obtained from the tachistoscopic study (Table 5) show that the experimental subjects reported a smaller number of words in all four categories as compared to normal readers. This difference, however, is

TABLE 5

Performance of subjects in the reading of different categories of words and nonwords

Subject	Computer presentation		Words correctly reported in tachistoscopic presentation			
	Nonwords Misread (max. 50)	Nonwords Misspelled (max. 50)	Nonword (max. 80)	Content word (max. 80)	Function word (max. 80)	CCC (max. 80)
S.H.	14	19	*	*	*	*
P.C.	11	14	32	53	49	20
O.C.	20	21	24	43	40	17
Controls (*n* = 3)	2	3	46	56	68	24

* S.H. was not administered the tachistoscopic task: the computer list was presented to S.H. without a computer.

most pronounced in the case of function words and pronunciable non-words. The greatest difference in the performance of the experimental and control subjects is seen in nonwords, with one subject (O.C.) reporting only half as many words as normal readers did. This finding is in agreement with a study by Frith (1978) which also found "spelling only retarded" subjects to be poor in reading nonwords.

The written spelling productions of the subjects were classified under three categories: phonologically unacceptable (e.g., *pouncil* → "poncil"), phonologically acceptable (e.g., *cade* → "kayed"), and real word substitution (e.g., *reng* → "rung"). The three subjects, S.H., P.C., and O.C., produced 19, 14, and 21 unacceptable spelling errors respectively; they also produced 29, 26, and 20 acceptable spellings and 2, 10, and 9 real words. The relative inability of these subjects to generate phonologically accurate spelling is obvious. The number of words spelled phonologically but inaccurately approximates the number of nonwords misread from the same list. The fact that all the subjects produced real words in spite of the definite instruction given that the stimuli were nonwords indicates that they may not be sensitive to the spelling of real words. Furthermore, these "errors" indicate that the subjects were not fully aware of alternative sound-letter relationships. For instance, while spelling "bace" as "base", the subject appears to feel constrained to use only the letter *s* for the /s/ sound; he (or she) appears not to be aware of the fact that the sound /s/ could also be represented by *c*. We believe that this inflexible adherence to the rudimentary "one sound-one letter" rule is a pervasive problem that underlies both reading and spelling difficulties of dyslexic subjects. In other words, these subjects are capable of phonetic transcription but are not adept at phonological transformation.

TASK 3: *Rate of reading.* The results of the studies so far discussed show that the three subjects with "pure spelling disability" show reading deficits similar to the ones seen in some developmental dyslexics. A question that naturally follows is: If they are poor readers why do these subjects appear to be normal readers? The data presented in Table 1 provide a clue. Even though their reading comprehension, as estimated by the Stanford Diagnostic Reading Test, is at college level their rate of reading falls far short of this standard. There appears to be a trade-off between speed and comprehension; these subjects may be able to comprehend written language by sacrificing speed. If this is true, their effective reading comprehension, which is a product of reading speed and comprehension, would be much lower than what the reading comprehension test scores indicate.

The reading rate of the subjects was determined by computing the speed with which they read a list of regular words (Coltheart, 1978) as well as three passages from the Stanford Diagnostic Reading Test.

Results. The number of words read per minute by the three subjects as well as members of the control group are shown in Table 6. Normal readers reportedly can read aloud connected prose at the rate of about 175 to 250 words per minute (Sticht, 1984). The data obtained by us for the control group are somewhat lower than this. Nevertheless, the difference in the reading speed between the experimental group and the normal readers is striking. This difference is more pronounced for isolated words in the list than for words in continuous text. The finding that the subjects are slow in reading isolated words rules out the possibility that extraneous factors such as eye movement could have contributed to their slow reading.

TABLE 6
Rate of reading (wpm): isolated words and continuous text

Subjects	Coltheart's list of regular words	Continuous text
S.H.	76.2	139.5
P.C.	67.6	123.3
O.C.	48.2	81.5
Controls	97.3	163.3

TASK 4: *Reading and spelling of regular and irregular words.* The subjects were asked to read aloud two lists of regular and irregular words matched for frequency and number of syllables (Coltheart, 1978). The words in each list were typed one below the other and each subject was asked to read them as quickly and as carefully as possible. The responses were taped. A week later, the same words were presented as a spelling test.

Results. As could be expected, the three subjects committed more errors in spelling than in reading (Table 7). Even though there was a tendency to misread more irregular words than regular words, the number of errors committed is too small to make any meaningful comparison. The

TABLE 7
Number of regular and irregular words misread and misspelled

Words	Reading (max. 36)*				Spelling (max. 36)			
	H.S.	P.C.	O.C.	Controls	H.S.	P.C.	O.C.	Controls
Regular	0	1	3	0	6	4	2	0.6
Irregular	0	2	5	0	10	8	8	1.3

* Three words from each list of the original 39 were accidentally left out.

subjects misspelled more irregular words than regular words and χ^2 test showed the differences to be significant at the 0.05 level.

Why did the subjects misspell more irregular than regular words? Before attempting to answer this question, it should be noted that the misspellings of some regular words indicate that the subjects do not possess a complete mastery of all the rules of spelling. This weakness is particularly apparent in the case of uncommon words, the spelling of which has to be generated by the application of pronunciation rules. Examples of such words are: *rub* → "rube"; *sort* → "sorte" (rule of final *e*); *biscuit* → "biskit", *circuit* → "circut", *treat* → "treet" (vowel digraphs). To return to the question raised at the beginning of this paragraph, misspellings of irregular words appear to be caused by three factors: (1) lack of complete mastery of rules of spelling as in the case of regular morphophonemes (e.g., *scarce* → "scarse", *gauge* → "gauze", *gross* → "grose"); (2) an attempt to conventionalize the spelling of irregular words (e.g., *sew* → "sow", *debt* → "dept", *bury* → "burry"); and (3) a tendency to substitute an unfamiliar word with a familiar one (e.g., *thorough* → "thrower", *trough* → "through", *borough* → "borrow"). A combination of poor mastery of grapheme-phoneme relational rules, word-familiarity effect, and a "conventionalization effect" contributes to the misspellings of a large number of irregular words. The spelling errors suggest that the subjects have rudimentary grapheme-phoneme relational skills but are not able to apply the more complex rules. In this respect, their spelling performance is similar to their reading performance.

TASK 5: *Reading of function words.* Information regarding the subjects' ability to read function words was derived from two sources: (1) the tachistoscopic study described in a previous section in which a set of four words was presented for a period of 500 milliseconds per set; and (2) from the subjects' performance on the reading of continuous text. The subjects were asked to read aloud the first three passages of the Stanford Diagnostic Reading Test and their reading was taped, transcribed, and analyzed.

Results. The performance of the subjects in reporting function words presented through the Tachistoscope is shown in Table 5. It can be seen that normal readers who were tested in the tachistoscopic task actually reported more function words than content words, a tendency which was reversed in the case of the three experimental subjects. The content vs. function-word discrepancy is a robust phenomenon observed consistently in developmental dyslexics (Aaron *et al.*, 1984).

Information regarding the subjects' performance of oral reading presented in Table 8 shows that they omitted or substituted more function words than content words. It is known that normal readers also have a tendency to omit and substitute function words while reading aloud but

TABLE 8

Errors committed by the three subjects in reading aloud continuous text

Subject	Function words and suffixes		Content words	
	Omission	*Substitution*	*Omission*	*Substitution*
S.H.	*at, the, for*	*is* → "was"	. . .	*director* → "editor"
	of, a	*the* → "a"		*compress* → "compass"
		on → "under"		*press* → "pass"
		about → "under"		
		an → "the"		
		the → "a"		
		for → "to"		
P.C.	*a* 3 (times)	*of* → "a"	sunny	*slip* → "skip"
	me (3 times)	*the* → "a"		
	of (2 times)	*while* → "will"		
	its (2 times)			
	out, to,			
	evening → "even"			
	reassured → "assured"			
O.C.	*also* → "so"	*can* → "may"		*guy* → "guide"
	subjected → "subject"	*build* → "built"		*cinch* → "clinch"
	gusts → "gust"			*bean* → "bee"
Total	22	12	1	7

such errors seldom reach the magnitude of misreading seen in the three experimental subjects. An interesting observation is that the target word and the substituted response word tend to belong to the same grammatical category; for instance, article *a* is substituted by another article *the*, verb *is* tends to be substituted by another verb *was*, the preposition *on* is read as *under*, and so on. These errors, therefore, appear to be the result of an over-reliance on context and may not be considered as visual errors. In this respect, function-word-reading errors differ from the content-word-reading errors which seem to be largely visual in nature. The mechanism responsible for the misreading of function words, therefore, may be different from the one responsible for content-word substitutions and in some way appears to be related to the "closed and open word" conceptualization.

5. DISCUSSION

The results of the analyses are summarized first. The three subjects show a consistent pattern of performance on all the tests given. In reading, the regularity or irregularity of the word has no marked effect. The frequency with which words appear in textbooks, however, has an effect on reading, with more errors being committed in the reading of low-frequency words. The subjects also make numerous mistakes in reading pronunciable nonwords. In addition, they make many substitution and omission errors of function words when reading continuous text. All the three subjects are also slow readers. As could be expected, they are all poor spellers. The regularity of the relationship of spelling to pronunciation affects spelling but not reading, with more irregular words being misspelled than regular words. Word frequency also affects spelling. Their spelling of nonwords shows that they are poor in generating phonologically acceptable spelling and that they are not fully aware of alternative letter-sound associations.

In a recently published report, Temple and Marshall (1983) provide a detailed description of a girl (H.M.) with developmental dyslexia. Since the symptoms presented by H.M. appear to be a virtual description of those of the three subjects reported in this paper, a summary of H.M.'s symptoms is presented here. Temple and Marshall describe H.M. in following terms: (a) average to above average intelligence, (b) oral vocabulary and speech normal, (c) great difficulty in reading nonwords, (d) majority of responses to nonwords result in real words, (e) reading unaffected by spelling to sound irregularity of the word, (f) poor performance in reading unfamiliar words, (g) erratic reading of function words in continuous text, (h) more errors committed in spelling irregular than regular words, and (i) majority of spelling errors were phonologically accurate. Temple and Marshall conclude that H.M. may be "confidently regarded as a developmental phonological dyslexic" (p. 517). Since S.H., P.C., and O.C. display virtually identical symptoms, they too can be considered as developmental phonologic dyslexics rather than as pure spelling retardates. The findings that these college students have subtle reading deficits is in conformity with a recently published study by Fischer *et al.* (1985) which compared 15 good spellers with 15 poor spellers from a college population. The study found that poor spellers were statistically inferior to good spellers both in oral reading and in the comprehension of printed text as assessed by the verbal aptitude score on the Scholastic Aptitude Test.

The subjects described in this study appear to have attained a reasonably good level of reading comprehension by relying excessively on the strategy of whole-word reading by sight. The following observations support such a possibility. Word regularity or irregularity does not have an appreciable effect on reading whereas word frequency does. Reading errors invariably result in a visually similar real word of higher frequency. Spelling errors show an erroneous parsing procedure which frequently results in familiar morphemes. Examples are: *legible* → "ledge ble"; *luncheon* → "lunch on"; *gentle* → "gen tel"; *benign* → "be nine"; *foreign* → "for gin". A number of investigators have proposed that an excessive dependence on spatial holistic strategy hinders the dyslexics' progress in reading (Aaron, 1978; Bakker *et al.*, 1976; Witelson, 1976). In discussing the paradoxical nature of specific spelling problems, Frith (1984) wonders about the "dissociation of such closely related skills as recognizing and reproducing a written word" (p. 83). She believes that the use of "partial cues" is sufficient for word recognition in reading whereas spelling requires a full-cue strategy. It is likely that reading by partial cues may not always work well with unfamiliar words. Jorm (1983), however, considers the "spelling only retardates" not to be deficient in reading single words. The present study shows that this statement may be true for familiar words but not for unfamiliar, low-frequency words.

The commonality between spelling and reading can also be defended on rational grounds. If "poor spellers but good readers" exist because reading and spelling are independent, separable processes, one can also expect to encounter "poor oral readers who are good spellers". This is what the principle of *double disassociation* would require. To our knowledge, no case of a "good speller but poor oral reader" has ever been reported in English-speaking subjects.

Furthermore, if the "spelling only retarded" subject is a good reader, why is he not able to read the word he has just written and recognize his own error and correct it by a process of trial and error? Simon and Simon (1973) refer to this as the "generate and test process" and consider it to be a reliable process that is used in spelling words. Consider a sample of misspellings produced by the three subjects in the spelling test: *charisma* → "crisma"; *gale* → "gal"; *rigid* → "ridget"; *foreign* → "forgin"; *gentle* → "gentel" *counsel* → "council"; *purchase* → "purchis"; *edges* → "edgis"; *damage* → "dammage"; *rating* → "ratting", etc. The pronunciation of each one of these misspelled word differs from that of the target word. If they could read correctly, the subjects could have detected their own errors and would have made efforts to improve the spelling.

Hatfield and Patterson (1983) give the following examples of their professional colleague's (R.P.) mispelling: *parents* → "per ants"; *whiskey* → "wis key". In addition to producing pronunciations that are different from the target words, the misspelled words also have different morphophonemic composition. Spelling errors of this kind would not arise if the subject can successfully pronunce the "nonwords" he wrote.

It was noted at the introductory section of this paper that a few neuropsychological reports of acquired dyslexia tend to support the view that reading and spelling are dissociable. The data used to assign these subjects to different subgroups of dyslexia and dysgraphia are, however, amenable to alternate interpretations. For instance, the oral reading of T.P. (Hatfield and Patterson, 1983) indicated that she was a surface dyslexic whereas her spelling errors were similar to the ones committed by phonological dyslexics thus suggesting a dissociation between reading and spelling. This interpretation was based on the observation that her written spelling of irregular words (from Coltheart's list) was worse than her spelling of regular words. The difficulty experienced by T.P. in spelling the "irregular" words, however, could be interpreted in another way. It was noted earlier (Table 2) that the correct spelling of words with vowel digraphs is mastered late in reading acquisition. Inspection of Coltheart's word-lists shows that there are more words with vowel digraphs in the irregular word-list than in the regular word-list, the actual numbers being 16 and 8. Thus, T.P.'s poor reading of the irregular words could also be due to an inability to use complex GPC rules because of phonological dyslexia and not due to a mechanical application of GPC rules. Another basis for describing T.P. as surface dysgraphic is that she made many errors in spelling homophonic words (e.g., sum → some). Many of her response words, however, had higher frequency than the test words. This renders a straightforward interpretation of these spelling errors difficulty since they would be attributed to phonological confusion as well as to frequency effect or a combination of the two. The developmental dyslexic, K.M., is described by Temple (1985b) as being neither a phonologic dyslexic nor a surface dyslexic; she was, however, classified as a surface dysgraphic on the supposition that reading and spelling are dissociable. It may, however, be noted that K.M. misread 5 out of 15 nonwords of 5—7 letters length thus suggesting some phonological difficulty. This is an unusually large number of errors for a 17-year-old girl who concentrated on English language and literature while in high school. K.M. is considered as surface dysgraphic since her spelling showed the regularity effect. As noted earlier, misspelling of irregular words could also be attributed to a failure to successfully use complex GPC rules in spelling thus leaving open the possibility that K.M. could be a case of phonological dysgraphic. In summary, it could be argued that both T.P. and K.M. are phonological dyslexics as well as phonological dysgraphics and that their reading and writing deficits are, therefore, parallel. This is not to say that dysgraphia subtypes do not exist (cf, Temple, 1986); it simply means that an incongruence reported between spelling and reading subtypes may be an artifact of classification.

The present study suggests that poor mastery of the phoneme-grapheme relational rules is associated with spelling difficulties. Since the three subjects described in the present study also have subtle deficits in reading, it may be speculated that poor mastery of the phoneme-grapheme relational skills is also responsible for their reading deficits. Since these subjects are mature adults with a number of years of education, it would appear that for proficient reading, the phonological mechanism (or route) is not merely optional but obligatory. Consideration of such a possibility, of course, depends upon whether reading and spelling are synergistic operations or not. Studies which claim that a direct semantic route alone is sufficient for reading have, for the most part, used evidence collected from lexical access tasks that use single words. Semantic decision tasks that utilize isolated test words may be ecologically one step removed from genuine reading process and may not enable the researcher to uncover subtle reading deficits that result from circumventing the indirect phonological route, especially when reading unfamiliar words and complex texts.

REFERENCES

Aaron, P. G.: 1978, 'Dyslexia, an imbalance in cerebral information processing strategies', *Perceptual and Motor Skills* **47**, 699—706.

Aaron, P. G.: 1989, *Dyslexia and Hyperlexia*, Kluwer, Dordrecht and Boston.

Aaron, P. G., Bommarito, T. G. and Baker, C.: 1984, 'The three phases of developmental dyslexia', in R. N. Malatesha and H. A. Whitaker (eds.), *Dyslexia: a Global Issue*, Martinus Nijhoff, The Hague.

Aaron, P. G., Olson, J. and Baker C.: 1985, 'The dyslexic college student: is he also dysphasic?', *Cognitive Neuropsychology* **2**, 115—147.

Bakker, D. J., Teunissen, J. and Bosch, J.: 1978, 'Development of laterality: reading patterns', in R. M. Knights and D. J. Bakker (eds.), *The Neuropsychology of Learning Disorders*, University Park Press, Baltimore, MD.

Baron, J., Treiman, R. M., Wilf, F. and Kellman, P.: 1980, 'Spelling and reading by rules', in U. Frith (ed.), *Cognitive Processes in Spelling*, Academic Press, London.

Beauvois, M. F. and Dérouesné, J.: 1979, 'Phonological Alexia: three dissociations', *Journal of Neurology, Neurosurgery, and Psychiatry* **42**, 115—124.

Beers, J. W.: 1980, 'Developmental strategies of spelling competence in primary school children', in E. H. Henderson and J. W. Beers (eds.), *Developmental and Cognitive Aspects of Learning to Spell*, International Reading Association, Newark, DE.

Bissex, G. L.: 1980, *Gnus at Wrk: A Child Learns to Write and Read*, Harvard Univ. Press, Cambridge, MA.

Bradley, L. and Bryant, P. E.: 1979, 'Independence of reading and spelling in backward and normal readers', *Developmental Medicine and Child Neurology* **21**, 504—514.

Bryant, P. E. and Bradley, L.: 1980, 'Why children sometimes write words which they do not read', in U. Frith (ed.), *Cognitive Processes in Spelling*, Academic Press, London.

Bradley, C. D., Garett, M. F. and Zurif, E. B.: 1980, 'Syntactic deficits in Broca's aphasia', in D. Caplan (ed.), *Biological Studies of Mental Processes*, The MIT Press, Cambridge, MA.

Bruskin, C. and Blank, M.: 1984, 'The effects of word class on children's reading and spelling', *Brain and Language* **21**, 219—232.

Calfee, R. C., Venezky, R. L. and Chapmen, R. S.: 1969, 'Pronunciation of synthetic words with predictable and unpredictable letter-sound correspondences', Technical Report, No. 11, Developmental Center for Cognitive Learning, Madison, Wisconsin.

Carroll, J. B., Davies, P. and Richman, B.: 1971, *Word Frequency Book*, Houghton Mifflin, New York.

Chomsky, C.: 1970, 'Reading, writing, and phonology', *Harvard Educational Review* **40**, 287—309.

Coltheart, M.: 1978, 'Lexical access in simple reading tasks', in J. Underwood (ed.), *Strategies of Information Processing*, Academic Press, New York.

Cook, L.: 1981, 'Misspelling analysis in dyslexia: observation of developmental strategy shifts', *Bulletin of the Orton Society* **3**, 123—134.

Dewey, G.: 1970, *Relative Frequency of English Spellings*, Teachers College Press, Columbia University, New York.

Fischer, F. W., Shankweiler, D. P. and Leiberman, I. Y.: 1985, 'Spelling proficiency and sensitivity to word structure', *Journal of Memory and Language* **24**, 423—441.

Frith, U.: 1978, 'From print to meaning and from print to sound or how to read without knowing how to spell', *Visible Language* **12**, 43—54.

Frith, U.: 1980, 'Unexpected spelling problems', in U. Frith (ed.), *Cognitive Processes in Spelling*, Academic Press, London.

Frith, U.: 1984, 'Specific spelling problems', in R. N. Malatesha and H. A. Whitaker (eds.), *Dyslexia: A Global Issue*, Martinus Nijhoff, The Hague.

Funnell, E.: 1983, 'Phonological processes in reading: new evidence from acquired dyslexia', *British Journal of Psychology* **74**, 159—180.

Gentry, J. R.: 1982, 'An analysis of developmental spelling in Gnys at Wrk', *The Reading Teacher* **36**, 192—200.

Gerber, M. M.: 1984, 'Orthographic problem-solving ability of learning disabled and normally achieving students', *Learning Disability Quarterly* **7**, 158—164.

Hatfield, F. and Patterson, K. E.: 1983, 'Phonological spelling', *Quarterly Journal of Experimental Psychology* **35A**, 451—468.

Jolly, H. B.: 1981, 'Teaching basic function words', *Reading Teacher* **35**, 136—140.

Jorm, A. F.: 1983, *The Psychology of Reading and Spelling Disabilities*, Routledge and Kegan Paul, London.

Karlsen, B., Madden, R. and Gardner, E. G.: 1974, *Stanford Diagnostic Reading Test*, Harcourt, Brace, and Jovanovich, New York.

Kean, M. L.: 1977, 'The linguistic interpretation of aphasic syndromes. Agrammatism in Broca's aphasia, an example', *Cognition* **5**, 9—46.

Margolin, D. I.: 1984, 'The neuropsychology of writing and spelling: semantic, phonological, motor, and perceptual processes', *Quarterly Journal of Experimental Psychology* **36A**, 459—489.

Marshall, J. C.: 1984, 'Toward a rational taxonomy of developmental dyslexia', in R. N. Malatesha and H. A. Whitaker (eds.), *Dyslexia: A Global Issue*, Martinus Nijhoff, The Hague.

Marshall, J. C. and Newcombe, F.: 1973, 'Patterns of paralexia: a psycholinguistic approach', *Journal of Psycholinguistic Research* **2**, 175—199.

Nelson, H. E.: 1980, 'Analysis of spelling errors in normal and dyslexic children', in U. Frith (ed.), *Cognitive Processes in Spelling*, Academic Press, London.

Nelson, H. E. and Warrington, E. K.: 1974, 'Developmental spelling retardation', *British Journal of Psychology* **65**, 265—274.

Nelson, H. E. and Warrington, E. K.: 1976, 'Developmental spelling retardation', in R. M. Knights and D. J. Bakker (eds.), *The Neuropsychology of Learning Disorders*, University Park Press, Baltimore, MD.

Perfetti, C. A. and Hogaboam, T.: 1975, 'Relationship between single word decoding and reading comprehension skills', *Journal of Educational Psychology* **67**, 461—469.

Read, C.: 1971, 'Preschool children's knowledge of English phonology', *Harvard Educational Review* **41**, 1—34.

Simon, D. P. and Simon, H. A.: 1973, 'Alternative uses of phonemic information in spelling', *Review of Educational Research* **43**, 115—137.

Snowling, M. J.: 1980, 'The development of grapheme-phoneme correspondence in normal and dyslexic readers', *Journal of Experimental Child Psychology* **29**, 294—305.

Spache, G.: 1940, 'Characteristic errors of good and poor readers', *Journal of Educational Research* **34**, 182—189.

Sticht, T. G.: 1984, 'Rate of comprehending by listening or reading', in J. Flood (ed.), *Understanding Reading Comprehension*, International Reading Association, Newark, DE.

Temple, C. M.: 1985a, 'Reading with partial phonology: developmental phonological dyslexia', *Journal of Psycholinguistic Research* **14**, 523—541.

Temple, C. M.: 1985b, 'Developmental surface dysgraphia: a case report', *Applied Psycholinguistics* **6**, 391—406.

Temple, C. M.: 1986, 'Developmental dysgraphias', *Quarterly Journal of Experimental Psychology* **38A**, 77—110.

Temple, C. M. and Marshall, J. C.: 1983, 'A case study of developmental phonological dyslexia', *British Journal of Psychology* **74**, 517—533.

Venezky, R.: 1970, *The Structure of English Orthography*, Mouton, The Hague.

Venezky, R.: 1976, *Theoretical and Experimental Base for Teaching Reading*, Mouton, The Hague.

Waters, G. S., Bruck, M. and Seidenberg, M.: 1985, 'Do children use similar processes to read and spell words?', *Journal of Experimental Child Psychology* **39**, 511—530.

Wijk, A.: 1966, *Rules of Pronunciation for the English Language: An Account of the Relationship between English Spelling and Pronunciation*, Oxford Univ. Press, London.

Witelson, S. F.: 1976, 'Abnormal right hemisphere specialization in developmental dyslexia', in R. M. Knight and D. J. Bakker (eds.), *The Neuropsychology of Learning Disorders*, University Park Press, Baltimore, MD.

APPENDIX

Words, Nonwords, and Subjects' Responses

Spelling-pronunciation rule	No.	High-frequency words	S.H.	P.C.	O.C.	Low-frequency words	S.H.	P.C.	O.C.	Pronounceable nonwords	S.H.	P.C.	O.C.
1. c = /k/	1	cake (244)				cape (22)				cade	cæd / cad	kayed	cage / cade
	2	cook (265)				coop (24)		cope					
	3	cabin (404)				center (3)							
	4	carbon (374)	claiburn			cadet (23)	cadete			cadlon	cadlun	cadlon	cadline
	5	local (286)				duct (3)				pocal	poocal / pokal	pokol	pokel
	6	picnic (128)				eclipse (31)	ealypse	eclispe	eipse				
	7	fraction (480)			fraction	escort (17)							
	8	doctor (406)				dictator (3)				mocton	mokten	mokin	mocken
2. c = /s/	9	cent (364)				cede (3)	sed			celt	celt	set / seat	seat
	10	central (287)				censor (2)		sensor		cept	sept	sept	sept
	11	circus (216)				centennial (2)	sentennial		centinal				
	12	citizen (230)	citisen	citizen		ceremonial (11)		ceremonial		cibly	sisybly	sibly	sibbly
	13	concern (250)			concen	secede (6)	succeed / succed	suceed	d.k. / secen	boncer	bouncer / bonser	bouncer / boncer	bouncer / bonzer
	14	council (200)	counsel			docile (6)				pouncil	pouncil	poncil	pasil / pongeel
	15	decided (200)				recital (4)		recitell		bace	bace	base	base
	16	decision (130)			decison	taciturn (2)	takituarn	d.k.	tactrun	crace	krace	crase	crase
3. ch = /k/	17	chord (303)	cord	cord	cord	chrome (13)			d.k. / chrom	chlor	slor / klore	clor / clor	clor

Appendix (continued)

Spelling-pronunciation rule	No.	High-frequency words	S.H.	P.C.	O.C.	Low-frequency words	S.H.	P.C.	O.C.	Pronunciable nonwords	S.H.	P.C.	O.C.
	18	chemical (376)				chorus (100)							
	19	character (242)	charector			charisma (2)	crisma	corse, chrisma	carisma				
	20	scholars (100)		scalars		echo (78)			eco				
	21	mechanic (131)			magnetic, mechic	monarchy (14)				brachy	breke	bresy, bracy	brachey
	22	technical (100)	technichal			alchemist (11)		chemist	d.k.	techan	tessan, tecon	techon	tacken
4. *ch* = /tʃ/	23	cheese (236)		cheeze		chap (2)				cheet	chet	cheat	sheet, cheat
	24	chamber (157)				chess (21)				chirk	chirp, chrp	chirp, chirp	chirp
	25	chosen (222)				charity (19)				choot	chute	short, choot	chute
	26	purchase (87)				bachelor (9)	bachiler	bachlor	bachler	nitcher	nitcher	nitcher	nitcher
	27	pitcher (114)				butcher (60)							
	28	machine (861)				luncheon (31)	lunchen	lunchon	lunchon	pachine	patch ue, pastion	passh ne, pachine	d.k., pachen
5. *g* = /g/	29	gift (200)				gale (27)	gail		gle				
	30	gate (267)				glare (36)				gake	g wk, gake	gake	g ge, gak
	31	globe (278)				gloss (8)				glone	glown	glone	glone
	32	gather (208)				garnet (39)			garment, gate				
	33	forget (314)				bogus (3)				logus	logus	logas	logas
	34	magnet (228)	magnut			magnate (0)	magnet	magnet		mignut	mignut	mignut	mignid
	35	regular (359)				migrate (35)		magnet	migret				

Appendix (continued)

Spelling-pronunciation rule	No.	High-frequency words	S.H.	P.C.	O.C.	Low-frequency words	S.H.	P.C.	O.C.	Pronunciable nonwords	S.H.	P.C.	O.C.
	36	flag (248)				brag (8)				plag	plegue / plague	plee / blag	plaegue / plag
6. g = /j/	37	germ (184)	genial			gems (18)	genius / gennus	genius		gern	gern	gern	grun
	38	gentle (200)		gental	gentel	genus (31)		genius	geus	gendal	gendel	gendle	gendle
	39	geology (109)	geollogy			generous (54)	gennirous			genks	janks	gurk	gerks
	40	generation (107)				generator (37)							
	41	caged (240)				rigid (49)	ridget	ridged	rigid				
	42	edges (269)	edgis			digit (2)	didget		diget	fedges	fedjes	fegigs	fledges / phegedes
	43	legend (141)	legion	ledgen		cogent (2)	cognet	cognent / cogen	d.k. / cognt	regend	ridgend	regon	rigun / regend
	44	religion (179)		religon		legible (10)	ledgable	ledgeble					
	45	stage (344)				merge (9)							
	46	range (351)				ledge (61)				mange	mange	manage / mange	mange / mange
7. g = /g/	47	damage (144)	dammage			manage (88)			magnet	fledge	fledge	fledge	phledge
	48	message (253)				porridge (21)	porrage	porrage					
	49	hanging (205)				linger (13)				signet	signet	signet	signid
	50	sang (264)				gang (81)				deng	deng	dang	deng
	51	string (483)				rating (20)	ratting			reng	reng	reng	rung
	52	hung (321)				prolong (6)							
8. g = /g/	53	sign (615)				assign (12)	assigne	asign	tign	tin / tine	tine	tine	signid
	54	design (487)	desine			resign (16)	resine			design	dln / dinn	dine	degaun / dine

Appendix (continued)

Spelling-pronunciation rule	No.	High-frequency words	S.H.	P.C.	O.C.	Low-frequency words	S.H.	P.C.	O.C.	Pronunciable nonwords	S.H.	P.C.	O.C.
	55	foreign (263)	forgine	forgin	foregn	benign (6)	benine	begin bennine	beign				
9. final *e*	56	not (18645)				rot (8)				kot	cute cout	kot	cute kot
	57	note (713)				rote (0)				kote	kout	koot	kot
	58	sit (549)				grip (46)				git	get git	gite git	git gedy
	59	site (108)				gripe (2)				gite	gite	guit	gite
	60	bar (325)				spar (13)			space	skar	scare skar	scar	scare scar
	61	bare (193)				spare (94)			spar	skare	skare	scare	skare
10. Secondary vowels "au"	62	aunt (3909)				auto (39)				ault	alt	alt	altez
	63	author (219)	auther			auction (18)				auro	arro	aro	aro
	64	august (150)				audible (9)	auddible	autobile	audiable				
	65	audience (209)			audiene	auxiliary (89)	augsillery		auxry				
	66	cause (508)				clause (91)		claus		faus	fose	fos	phoss
	67	pause (109)				haul (53)	hale			kaul	cowel	call	call
	68	launch (100)			lanch	haunt (5)							
	69	daughter (288)				applause			aplause				
11. *ui* =	70	fruit (459)		friuit		bruise (29)	bruse			bruit	brewt	brute	brlt brute
	71	build (857)				biscuit (62)		biskit	buicuit	miscuit	misket	miskit	miscet
	72	require (300)				acquire (33)	acquire	aquire	acire				

Appendix (continued)

Spelling-pronunciation rule	No.	High-frequency words	S.H.	P.C.	O.C.	Low-frequency words	S.H.	P.C.	O.C.	Pronunciable nonwords	S.H.	P.C.	O.C.
12. *ou* =	73	suitable (143)				recruit (10)	*recrute*						
	74	ought (220)				ounce (48)				ounch	*ounce* *ounch*	*ounce* *once*	*onch*
	75	rough (292)				clout (4)				pough	*pauf*	*pause* *puff*	*poach* *poff*
Totals	75					75				50			

Words underlined are oral responses.
Words in italic are written spellings.
Figures in parenthesis represent word frequency.
Correct responses for real words are not shown.
d.k. = don't know.

BEVERLY D. K. MAUL AND LINNEA C. EHRI

MEMORY FOR SPELLINGS IN NORMAL AND DYSGRAPHIC SPELLERS

Do Dysgraphics Spell by Ear but not Eye?

The ability to spell is highly correlated with the ability to read. Shanahan (1984) reported correlations of 0.66 and 0.60 in samples of second and sixth graders, respectively. Various reasons for the high correlations can be identified. One is that some of the same knowledge sources, processes and strategies are utilized (Ehri, 1986; Simon and Simon, 1973; Simon, 1976). In order to read and spell words whose spellings are familiar, people are thought to access letter-analyzed representations of specific words stored in lexical memory. Lexical memory for specific words spellings can also be used to read and spell unfamiliar words by analogy, that is, by retrieving from memory words that resemble the unfamiliar words either in spelling pattern or in pronunciation, for example, reading or spelling "grief" by analogy to "brief" (Marsh *et al.*, 1980). Another way to read and spell unfamiliar words is to utilize one's general knowledge of the orthographic system which includes grapheme—phoneme and pho-neme—grapheme relations, letter position constraints, and morphophon-emic and morphographic spellings patterns (Becker *et al.*, 1980; Venezky, 1970).

A second explanation for the high correlation between reading and spelling is that reading is the primary way that people learn correct spellings of specific words. Readers see many more words in their reading than they ever practice in their writing. Good readers read more than poor readers so they are exposed to the correct spellings of many more words and hence learn them better. In English, exposure to words is essential for learning their correct spellings because many of the spellings are variable and hard to predict on the basis of general knowledge of the spelling system (Hanna *et al.*, 1986).

Although reading and spelling are highly correlated, the correlation is not perfect, very likely because the processes used to read and spell are not identical. The process of reading words involves simply recognizing which words in a reader's lexicon are symbolized by those particular letter sequences whereas the process of spelling words involves recalling entire letter sequences. Recognition is known to be an easier process than recall. Moreover, word reading can be conducted effectively with partial knowl-edge of letters, particularly when the context provides syntactic and semantic information about words as well (e.g., "In the jungle, the el_ph_t . . ."). In contrast, the process of spelling words perfectly requires com-plete knowledge of letters in words. Because word spellings in English are

R. M. Joshi (ed.), Written Language Disorders, 25—42.
© 1991 *Kluwer Academic Publishers. Printed in the Netherlands.*

difficult to predict, it is necessary to have all of a word's letters stored in memory in order to spell the word perfectly.

Another difference that makes reading easier involves the transforming process between print and speech (Cronnell, 1978). In reading, letters are transformed into sounds whereas, in spelling, sounds are transformed into letters. In English there are approximately 40 distinctive sounds but about 70 letters or letter combinations to symbolize these sounds. As a result, producing correct pronunciations of letters is more probable than producing correct spellings for pronunciations because there are fewer options in the former case. For example, the letter K in a word is almost always pronounced /k/ whereas the sound /k/ may be spelled in at least six different ways: K, C, CK, Q, X, and CH. Another factor making reading easier is that units in the stimulus word are more apparent in the case of print (i.e., letters) than in the case of pronunciations where constituent phonemes are abstract, overlapping, and not directly represented in the speech stream (Liberman *et al.,* 1967).

Given these differences between reading and spelling processes, it is not surprising to find a few reader/spellers who are exceptions to the rule. Frith (1978, 1979, 1980, 1983) has studied people who exhibit disparities in their reading and spelling skills in English. In looking for subjects, she found no people who were adequate spellers but poor readers, indicating that spelling skill does not develop in the absence of reading skill in English. However, she found a small number of people above the age of 10—11 who had adequate reading skill but poor spelling skill. She called these people *dysgraphics* or unexpectedly poor spellers.

To explore the reading and spelling capabilities of dysgraphics, Frith (1978, 1980) compared them to two other groups of spellers: people who could read and comprehend text as well as dysgraphics but were much better at spelling English words correctly, whom we shall call *normals,* and people who were as poor at spelling words as dysgraphics but in contrast were much poorer in reading comprehension than dysgraphics, referred to as *dyslexics.* Frith examined subjects' ability to generate plausible phonetic spellings of nonsense words and found that dysgraphics performed almost as well as the normal spellers and much better than the dyslexics. She concluded that dysgraphics are not deviant in their ability to generate phonetic spellings of words. Rather dysgraphics' primary difficulty is in remembering the correct spellings of real words, many of which are not completely phonetic. Frith also examined subjects' reading skills and found that dysgraphics were comparable to normal spellers in being able to convert familiar printed words into meanings but were deficient in their ability to convert unfamiliar print to speech, as indicated on tasks that required reading aloud, judging rhymes, and reading nonsense words. Frith (1980) concluded that the processes used by normal spellers to read and spell are more similar than the processes used by dysgraphics. Whereas normals read and spell words by ear as well as by eye, that is, by sight-word memory as well as by print-speech conversion, dysgraphics read words by eye and they spell words by ear.

The purpose of the present study was to investigate whether the transfer from word reading to word spelling is greater among normal spellers than among dysgraphics, as Frith suggests. It was reasoned that if normals use the same processes to read and to spell words whereas dysgraphics use different processes, then manipulation of the word-reading task ought to have a greater impact upon the spelling performance of normal spellers than upon that of dysgraphics. One way to manipulate the word-reading task so that it has an impact upon subjects' ability to spell the words they read is to have subjects either read the words aloud on a list or read the words silently in the context of a story. We know from previous research that readers remember the spellings of unfamiliar words better if they read them in isolation on a list than if they read them in sentence contexts (Ehri and Roberts, 1979, Ehri and Wilce, 1980). Also we would expect that readers' memory for spellings would be better if they read the words aloud than if they read them silently because the former task requires greater attention to letters than the latter task. This was the manipulation used in the present study.

We selected eighth and ninth graders who were matched in reading comprehension ability (all above average) but who differed in word-spelling skill, with normal spellers above average and dysgraphics well below average. Subjects were first taught orally the meanings and pronunciations of 15 target words and then were exposed to the words' spellings in one of two types of reading tasks. Half of the normals and dysgraphics were shown the target words on a list which they read aloud. The other half were shown the target words in a story which they read silently. Then subjects' memory for the spellings of the words was measured with a dictation task and a recognition task.

We expected that subjects who read target words orally in isolation would remember the spellings better than subjects who read the words silently in context. More importantly, we expected that if dysgraphics use different strategies to read and to spell words whereas normals use the same strategy, then the impact of the reading manipulation on spelling skill ought to be minimal for dysgraphics but substantial for normals. That is, we ought to see an interaction between reading treatment and spelling ability group. Normal spellers' memory for spellings ought to increase substantially when they read words in isolation rather than in context whereas dysgraphics' memory for spellings ought to increase only minimally.

1. METHOD

1.1. *Subjects*

The subjects were 36 eighth and 32 ninth graders (35 males, 33 females) attending two junior high schools in a suburban agricultural community. Their mean age was 172.1 months (14 years). All subjects were better-than-average readers as measured by the reading comprehension subtest of the Comprehensive Test of Basic Skills (CTBS).

To select these subjects, we identified students whose CTBS reading comprehension scores were above the 57th percentile and whose CTBS spelling scores were either above the 55th percentile or below the 44th percentile. Reading comprehension scores were used to form matched pairs of normal and dysgraphic spellers within each grade. To verify that subjects met these criteria, scores on a second reading comprehension test and spelling test were obtained and used to eliminate subjects scoring too high or too low. Of the 106 students originally selected, 14 were eliminated by second test scores and 24 failed to return parental consent forms. The final sample consisted of 34 pairs of students. The mean reading comprehension percentile scores of the two groups on the first test were 76.6 (normal spellers) vs. 76.5 (dysgraphic spellers), on the second test 75.9 (normal) vs. 73.2 (dysgraphic). The mean spelling percentile scores on the first test were 79.2 (normal) vs. 31.1 (dysgraphic) and on the second test were 81.7 (normal) vs. 27.5 (dysgraphic). The two groups were very similar in age, 171 months (normal) vs. 173 months (dysgraphic). Matched-pair t-tests revealed that only the spelling means differed statistically ($p < 0.01$), not the other means ($p > 0.05$). The presence of spelling differences and the absence of comprehension differences between normal and dysgraphic spellers on the second tests enhance confidence that normals and dysgraphics were truly different in spelling but not in reading comprehension skill.

1.2. *Materials*

Fifteen words whose spellings and meanings were thought to be unfamiliar to junior high students were selected as target words. These are listed in Table 1. Definitions of the words were written and also a story containing all of the words. In one version of the story, the target words each appeared once. In another version, three of the target words were repeated. The story was about the luxurious life of a Roman emperor's horse. Three questions, each having two-point answers, were written to test comprehension of the story. A spelling recognition test was created consisting of the target words correctly spelled plus three misspellings of each target word. A nonsense word reading task was designed to test subjects' phonological

TABLE 1

Spellings and pronounciations of target words; letter categories score in the spelling post-test

Standard spelling	Pronunciation	Schwa letters	Silent letters	Double letters
Caligula	/kə lig′ yə lə/	a u a		
Frosinone	/frō sə nōn′/	i	e	
Incitatus	/in sə tā′ təs/	i u		
Vesuvius	/və soo′ vē əs/	e u		
Apennines	/a pə nīnz′/	e	e	nn
seismic	/sīz′ mik/		e	
crystalline	/kris′ tə lin/	a	e	ll
incessantly	/in ses′ ənt lē/	a		ss
cantatas	/kən tä′ təz/	a a		
banishment	/ban′ ish mənt/	e		
virtually	/vûr choo ə lē/	e	a	ll
Consullar	/kon′ sə lər/	u a		ll
Commodus	/ko′ mə dəs/	o u		mm
equinal	/ē kwīn′ əl/	a		
horrendous	/hô ren′ dəs/	u	o	rr
Total number		21	6	7

recoding skill. It consisted of 10 nonsense words: enstrector; glispliness; flouretable; spighter; phonoctiary; lampaign; wrentlesome; reblouthing; precile; fileage.

1.3. *Procedures and Design*

Members of subject pairs were assigned randomly, one to a treatment in which subjects were exposed to the spellings of target words on a list which they read aloud, the other to a treatment in which subjects were exposed to target spellings in a story that they read silently. Subjects were tested individually. Tasks were administered in one session lasting about 40 minutes.

First, all subjects were taught orally the meanings of the 15 target words, five words at a time. The experimenter defined each word and the subject repeated the word. For example, "When someone does something incessantly, he does it without stopping. Say 'incessantly'." Then she quizzed subjects about the words by repeating questions in varying orders until all five were answered correctly with the target word. For example, "What word means doing something without stopping?"

After pronunciations and meanings of the three sets of words had been mastered, the experimental treatment began. Half of the subjects were shown the target words printed on a list and were told to read each word carefully out loud. The other subjects were given a story containing the words and were told to read the story silently and to pay attention to its meaning because they would be asked some questions about the story later. Story-reading subjects indicated that they were finished by closing the folder containing the story.

Following the treatments, subjects performed two spelling tasks. In the spelling production task, the experimenter pronounced each target word once and subjects wrote it. In the spelling recognition task, subjects circled the spelling they thought was correct. After this, subjects in the context condition were tested for their comprehension of the story.

In the final task, subjects phonologically recoded 10 nonsense words. Five of the words were considered to have only one correct pronunciation, five could be pronounced in one of two ways.

The procedures used to test subjects in the context condition differed slightly at the two schools. At one school, eight normals and eight dysgraphics read the version of the story that had no target words repeated, and they took the spelling tests before the comprehension tests. At the other school, nine normals and nine dysgraphics read the version of the story that had three target words repeated, and they took the comprehension test before the spelling tests. Thus, subjects at one school saw three of the words fewer times and took and spelling test sooner after reading the words than subjects at the other school.

2. RESULTS

2.1. Pretests

To compare the various subject and treatment groups, ANOVAs were conducted. The independent variables were spelling skill (normal vs. dysgraphic) and word-reading treatment (isolation vs. context). To verify that the four groups (NI, — normal spellers reading isolated words; DI, — dysgraphic spellers reading isolated words, NC, — normals reading words in contexts; DC, dysgraphics reading words in contexts) did not differ pre-experimentally in any respect except spelling skill, two-way ANOVAs were conducted on pretest scores (i.e., CTBS spelling scores, CTBS reading comprehension scores, age). The only effect to reach statistical significance was the difference in spelling skill. Normal spellers out performed dysgraphics ($p < 0.01$). No other main effects or interactions were significant (all p's > 0.05).

Prior to reading the words, all subjects learned their pronunciations and meanings. To determine whether the groups differed in the number of times the sets of five definitional questions had to be repeated before all were answered correctly, an ANOVA was conducted. Means did not differ statistically, all F's < 1, $M = 11.2$ repetitions (NI), 11.1 (DI), 10.9

(NC), 11.6 (DC), $MSE = 8.33$. This indicates that the normal and dysgraphic spellers did not differ in how quickly they learned to say the target words and recognize their definitions.

2.2. *Spelling Post-tests*

The main purpose of this study was to determine whether normal spellers' memory for spellings would be more affected by the way they read the words than dysgraphics' memory for spellings. To assess these effects, ANOVAs were conducted on performances in the spelling tasks. The independent variables were spelling skill and reading treatment. Several dependent measures were analyzed: number of words spelled perfectly; number of letters correct; numbers of specific types of letters correct (double letters, silent letters, schwa letters; see lists in Table 1); number of spellings correctly distinguished in the recognition task.

Not surprisingly, normal spellers performed significantly better than dysgraphic spellers on all of these measures. F-values ranged from 31.61 (double letters correct) to 119.12 (words spelled perfectly), $df = 1, 64$, all p's < 0.01. Normal spellers wrote 46% of the words correctly, dysgraphics wrote 20% (15 words total). Normals wrote 90% of the letters correctly, dysgraphics 81% (135 letters total). Normals recognized 67% of the correct spellings on the recognition test, dysgraphics 45% (15 words total).

Subjects who read words in isolation outperformed subjects who read words in context on all measures but the schwa letter measure:

> $M = 5.8$ vs. 4.1 words spelled correctly (maximum 15),
> $F(1, 64) = 23.44, p < 0.01$;
> $M = 117$ vs. 114 letters correct (maximum 135),
> $F(1, 64) = 5.61, p < 0.05$;
> $M = 3.4$ vs. 2.2 double letters correct (maximum 7),
> $F(1, 64) = 15.49, p < 0.01$;
> $M = 4.7$ vs. 3.6 silent letters correct (maximum 6),
> $F(1, 64) = 18.49, p < 0.01$;
> $M = 13.0$ vs. 12.1 schwa letters correct (maximum 21),
> $F(1, 64) = 2.01, p > 0.05$;
> $M = 8.8$ vs. 7.9 words recognized correctly (maximum 15),
> $F(1, 64) = 4.21, p < 0.05$.

This confirmed our expectation that the experience of reading words aloud in isolation develops better memory for spellings than the experience of reading words silently in a story.

Our main prediction was that significant interactions would be detected between reading experience and spelling skill, specifically, that reading experience would influence the spelling memory of normal spellers more than that of dysgraphics. Results are portrayed in Figure 1. In the ANOVAs, interactions on five out of six measures were not significant, p's > 0.05. As evidenced in Figure 1 by the parallel slopes, dysgraphics improved their word spellings to the same extent as normal spellers when they read words in isolation rather than in context. This indicates that reading processes transfer to spelling among dysgraphics as well as among normals and to the same extent.

The one interaction that reached significance involved memory for double letters, $F(1, 64) = 8.99$, $p < 0.01$. However, the pattern of mean recall scores was the opposite of that expected. As evident in Figure 1, dysgraphics remembered many more double letters when they read words aloud in isolation than when they read words silently in context whereas normal spellers remembered only slightly more in isolation. This finding indicates that dysgraphics' spelling of double letters is more, not less dependent upon reading experiences than that of normal spellers.

We sought evidence for Frith's claim in another way. Based on the observation that spelling recognition performance is more like word reading performance than spelling production performance, we thought that dysgraphics might find the visual information that they gained from reading words relatively more useful for recognizing correct spellings on the multiple choice task than for producing correct spellings on the dictation task, whereas normals might find their visual knowledge equally useful on both tasks. If true, then we ought to observe an interaction between spelling ability groups and spelling tasks. Specifically, spelling recognition performance ought to surpass spelling production perform-ance more among dysgraphics than among normals. To test this hypothe-sis, a three-way ANOVA was conducted with reading treatment, spelling

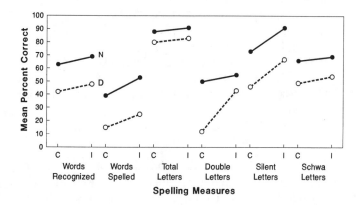

Fig. 1. Mean percent words and letters spelled correctly in the spelling post-tests as a function of reading treatment (C = context, I = isolation) and speller skill group (N = normal spellers, D = dysgraphic spellers).

skill, and spelling task as the independent variables. The dependent measure was number of words correct. Main effects of all three variables were significant (all p's < 0.01). (Main effects of spelling skill and reading treatment have already been described.) Subjects recognized more correct spellings than they produced, $F(1, 64) = 246.49$, $p < 0.01$. However, the interaction between spelling task and spelling skill fell short of significance, $F(1, 64) = 2.84$, $0.05 < p < 0.10$. Dysgraphics recognized a mean of 3.8 more words than they spelled correctly, and normal spellers recognized a mean of 3.1 more words than they spelled.

These findings along with those above fail to support Frith's (1978, 1980) claim that dysgraphics contrast with normal spellers in using different processes to read words and to produce their spellings. Rather results indicate that the visual information retained about words by reading them is accessed by dysgraphics as well as normals to spell the words.

It is interesting to note how well dysgraphics remembered unpredictable letters in the spellings of specific words after reading them. Figure 1 shows that after reading words in isolation, dysgraphics recalled 43% of the double letters and 67% of the silent letters. These are letters that presumably could not be guessed correctly by using a phonetic spelling strategy and so have to be remembered.[1] These findings clearly show that dysgraphics do not spell strictly by ear but also access visual information about letters acquired from their reading experiences to spell.

In a previous study (Drake and Ehri, 1984), it was noticed that good and poor spellers differed more in their memory for completely correct spellings of words than in their memory for correct letters in the spellings. A similar pattern was evident in the present study. Normal spellers recalled 90% of the letters correctly but only 46% of the words; dysgraphics recalled 81% of the letters, but only 20% of the words. The difference in recall favoring normals over dysgraphics was only 9% for letters but 26% for words. To verify the statistical significance of this interaction, the proportions of words and letters correctly spelled were calculated for each subject and a three-way ANOVA was conducted. The independent variables were spelling skill, reading treatment, and spelling unit (words vs. letters). The interaction between spelling skill and spelling unit was significant, $F(1, 64) = 92.86$, $p < 0.01$. These results indicate that dysgraphics are almost as good at producing correct letters as normal spellers. Where they are weak relative to normal spellers is in their ability to produce entirely correct spellings. This suggests that spelling processes at the word level rather than at the letter level are central in accounting for dysgraphics' spelling disability.

In the ANOVA comparing the proportions of words and letters spelled correctly, the interaction between reading treatment and spelling unit was also significant, $F(1, 64) = 22.10$, $p < 0.01$. Comparison of slopes in

Figure 1 reveals that the increase in spelling performance occurring when words were read in isolation rather than in context was much greater on the word measure than on the letter measure. Whereas the mean proportion of letters spelled correctly increased from 27% to 39%, the mean proportion of words spelled correctly increased from 84% to 86%. This indicates that the boost given to memory by reading spellings aloud operated at the lexical level more than at the single letter level. However, as evident in Figure 1, double and silent letters exhibited a substantial boost from the reading treatment as well, indicating that not all letters fit this pattern. One explanation may have to do with how spellings were produced. It may be that the strategy of generating phonetically plausible spellings of the words enabled subjects to compensate for their lack of memory for correct spellings. This strategy would be expected to mitigate effects of reading treatment more on the letter measure than on the word measure because more of the letters could be guessed accurately using this strategy, all letters, that is, except double and silent letters.

Frith (1980) found that dysgraphics were as skilled as normal spellers in producing phonetically plausible spellings of nonsense words. In the present study, we calculated the proportion of misspellings that were acceptable phonetic forms. Mean values were 66% for dysgraphics and 74% for normals. The difference was not significant statistically, $F(1, 64) = 2.36$, $p > 0.05$. These results replicate Frith's finding. In absolute terms, dysgraphics produced a mean of only three conventionally correct spellings but a mean of 10.8 phonetically acceptable spellings (maximum 15), indicating that the majority of their spellings though wrong were phonetically accurate.

2.3. *Reading Tasks*

Frith (1978, 1980) found that dysgraphics were poorer at decoding nonsense words than normal spellers. To assess this relationship in the present study, performances in the nonsense word decoding task were compared. The ANOVA revealed that dysgraphics pronounced significantly fewer words correctly than normals, $M = 5.5$ vs. 7.3 correct (10 maximum), $F(1, 64) = 22.22$, $p < 0.01$, hence corroborating Frith's finding.

Dysgraphics also pronounced fewer target words correctly than normal spellers when they were required to read them aloud during the isolation reading treatment. An ANOVA comparing the mean numbers of target words read correctly showed that dysgraphics performed significantly worse than normals, $M = 8.8$ vs. 11.3 words correct (15 maximum), $F(1, 32) = 12.58$, $p < 0.01$. It was not the case that dysgraphics erred more because they expended less effort decoding target words. An ANOVA of the time spent in this task revealed that dysgraphics spent significantly more time looking at the words and attempting to read them than normals, $M = 1.56$ vs. 1.24 minutes, $F(1, 32) = 4.72$, $p < 0.05$. Inspection of their readings revealed that dysgraphics gave every word a pronunciation that resembled the correct form, indicating that they were exposed sufficiently to each spelling and recognized which word it was symbolizing. These observations rule out the possibility that dysgraphics remembered fewer spellings because they did not study them as much. In fact, timewise they studied them more. Two reasons might explain why dysgraphics had more trouble than normals reading the target words that both groups had just learned orally equally well. Either dysgraphics forgot more pronunciations than normals, or they had more trouble matching up the pronunciations they knew to the spellings they saw. The latter difficulty might be expected given dysgraphics' weaker phonological recoding skill.

In the context treatment, subjects read the story containing the target words silently. Dysgraphics spent slightly more time reading the story than normals, $M = 2.08$ vs. 1.81 minutes, although the difference failed to reach significance, $F(1, 32) = 3.33$, $0.05 < p < 0.10$. It was not the case that dysgraphics skipped over words and did not read the story as accurately. In the ANOVA of scores on the reading comprehension test, dysgraphics answered as many questions correctly as normals, $M = 4.6$ correct (dysgraphics) vs. 4.3 correct (normals) (6 maximum), $F(1, 32) = 1.24$, $p > 0.05$. This is further evidence that the two groups did not differ in reading comprehension ability.

2.4. Effects of Change in the Experimental Procedures

Midway through the study when the experimenter moved to the second junior high school to test subjects, two procedures in the context reading treatment were changed. Repetition of three target words in the story (i.e., proper names: Caligula, Incitatus, Frosinone) was eliminated and other nouns or pronouns were substituted for these words. Also, the spelling tests were moved ahead of the comprehension questions so that subjects spelled words right after they read the story. To determine whether these changes affected performance, t-tests were conducted on spelling and comprehension measures to compare subjects in the context condition at the two schools. One difference reached significance. Students who answered comprehension questions right after they read the story recalled more information than students who waited until after the spelling tests to complete the comprehension test, $M = 4.9$ vs. 4.0 correct, $t(32) = 2.66$, $p < 0.05$. Although delaying the comprehension test impaired comprehension performance, delaying the spelling tests until after the comprehension test had no effect on spelling recall. The mean numbers of words spelled perfectly, letters recalled, and spellings recognized correctly by the two groups did not differ statistically (all p's > 0.05). These findings show that whether subjects read all of the words once and spelled words right after reading the story or whether they read three words more than once and took the spelling tests after a slight delay did not effect their overall spelling scores. Perhaps taking the spelling test sooner after exposure to the words compensated for seeing the words only once. A t-test applied to the mean times taken to read the passage indicated that the word repetition variable did not affect reading time ($p > 0.05$). In sum, these results indicate that the procedural changes were minor and had no effect upon spelling performances.

3. DISCUSSION

The primary purpose of this study was to seek evidence for the claim that dysgraphic spellers contrast with normal spellers in using different processes to read and spell, the eye to read and the ear to spell. The approach taken was to manipulate dysgraphic and normal spellers' reading experiences with words in a way that should influence their ability to spell the words if reading transfers to spelling. We reasoned that if the claim is true, then the reading manipulation should exert less influence on dysgraphics' ability to spell the words than upon normals' word spelling ability. Results failed to yield the expected interaction. The reading manipulation was successful in influencing dysgraphic and normal subjects' ability to spell the words they read to the same extent, with words read aloud in isolation spelled better than words read silently in context. In fact, on one measure, dysgraphics were affected *more* than normal spellers, not the reverse. Dysgraphics' memory for double letters increased more than normal spellers' memory when the task was switched from reading words in context to reading words in isolation. This differential increase was not due to ceiling effects on the measure. These results indicate that processes used by dysgraphics to read words do transfer and influence their ability to spell the words, to the same extent as happens with normal spellers.

The fact that dysgraphics were moderately successful at recalling double letters and silent letters correctly is clear evidence that dysgraphics spell words by accessing visual information they have gained by reading the words. Because these letters cannot be guessed by spelling words phonetically, if readers spell them correctly, it must be because they store them in memory from their reading experiences.

In order to explain present findings, it is important to review how subjects spell words whose printed forms are familiar (Ehri, 1986; Simon, 1976; Simon and Simon, 1973). Spellers are thought to access lexical memory for information about letters in the spellings of specific words they have read or spelled before. If all of the information is there, it is retrieved and the spelling is produced. If some or all of the information is missing, then the speller uses his/her knowledge of the orthographic system to generate a plausible spelling or to fill in missing parts with a plausible spelling. Present findings indicate that when people read words, they do retain information about their spellings in lexical memory, and this information is used to produce as well as to recognize correct spellings of the words. Dysgraphics as well as normal spellers retain information about spellings when they read words, and they access this information to spell the words. However, present findings also show that dysgraphics remember less about spellings from their reading than normals. As a result, they are forced to generate more parts missing in memory than normal spellers. Because dysgraphics' knowledge of the spelling system is primarily phonetic, they end up spelling words they have forgotten either partially or completely by ear.

Given that our dysgraphic subjects were very poor spellers, it is perhaps surprising that they produced so many correct letters in the spellings, 80—83% (see Figure 1). One explanation is that they were able to guess many of the letters correctly because they generated plausible phonetic spellings of the words. Another explanation is that they were able to store many of the letters in lexical memory. According to our theory of spelling acquisition (Drake and Ehri, 1984; Ehri, 1980, 1984, 1987, in press; Ehri and Wilce, 1979, 1980b, 1982, 1986), spellers retain information from their reading to spell words by processing letters as symbols for sounds detected in pronunciations and by storing these associations in memory. This enables spellers to remember phonetic letters. In addition, if they create spelling pronunciations of words that include sounds for silent and nondistinctively pronounced letters (i.e., schwa), this may enable them to remember these letters as well (Drake and Ehri, 1984). Because dysgraphics know basic grapheme—phoneme relations, they should be able to store and retrieve letters from lexical memory in this way. It is interesting to note that most dysgraphics spelled at least as many letters as were phonetic. Adopting a set of phoneme—grapheme rules that captured the most common regularities,[2] we were able to account for 75% of the letters. Inspection of individual scores among dysgraphics revealed that the proportions of correct letters ranged from 74% to 91%. Moreover, two-thirds of the scores were at or above 80% correct. This reveals that the majority of the dysgraphics were remembering or generating most of the phonetic letters plus some of the nonphonetic letters.

Dysgraphics produced correctly almost as many letters as normal spellers, but they were substantially worse at spelling words correctly. Very likely the reason is that normal spellers possess more sophisticated knowledge about the spelling system than dysgraphics, and they use this knowledge both to store more complete spellings of words in memory from their reading as well as to generate better guesses about spellings. In addition to letter-sound correspondences, they know morphophonemic rules, morphographic spellings, and spelling patterns common to many words (Becker *et al.*, 1980; Marsh *et al.*, 1981; Venezky, 1970). Also, because normals know complete spellings of words, they are better at recognizing analogous word spellings (Marsh *et al.*, 1980). Frith (1980) found that normal spellers were more apt to spell words by analogy than dysgraphics.

Although we have shown that reading transfers to spelling in dysgraphics, Frith might find fault with our experiment. She might argue that we caused dysgraphics to read the words in ways that they do not normally use when they read words on their own and that our manipulations were the reason why their spelling performance mirrored that of normal readers. By requiring dysgraphics to read the target words aloud, we forced a phonological recoding strategy upon them. By teaching dysgraphics the meanings of target words before they read them in the story, we made them more interested in the words and hence more likely to notice their spellings when they read the story silently. Whether these possibilities are valid awaits further study.

Another possible limitation of our study is that the effect of dysgraphics' reading on their spelling might be limited to their short-term memory and might not persist into long-term memory. We do not know whether this is true because our spelling tests were given right after the reading task, not after a delay. This possibility needs to be studied. However, even if it is true that dysgraphics do not remember spellings of words they have read for very long, this still does not invalidate our finding that dysgraphics spell by eye in some circumstances and, moreover, that they have access to visual information when they spell. In this respect, it cannot be claimed that dysgraphics spell only by ear.

One explanation why readers may not store the spellings of words in memory as effectively when they read the words silently in context rather than orally in lists is that readers use context cues to anticipate words, they slight attention to letters when they recognize from a few letters that the expected words are present, and they do not convert spellings into pronunciations because this is not needed to perform the silent reading task. Stanovich (1980, 1986) among others has found that poor readers are more apt than good readers to compensate by relying on context to recognize words because their decoding skills are weak and not automatic. One might expect that dysgraphics would also compensate more than normal spellers when they read words silently in text because dysgraphics are weaker decoders. However, evidence bearing on this hypothesis was mostly negative in the present study. Memory for spellings did not decline more for dysgraphics than for normals when the spellings were read in context than when they were read in isolation except on one measure, that involving memory for double letters. Thus, only very limited evidence was obtained indicating that dysgraphics slight letter cues more than normal spellers in their silent reading as contrasted to their oral reading. However, as indicated above, it may be that our findings do not reflect what dysgraphics normally do when they read text silently. In our study, dysgraphics' attention may have been drawn to target words in stories because the target words had just been taught orally, hence heightening their interest in the words' spellings.

One methodological weakness of studies comparing dysgraphic and normal spellers is that often no steps are taken to combat effects of regression to the mean. This problem arises when two variables that are highly correlated (e.g., reading and spelling skill) are used to form subject groups by selecting people whose scores are similar on one variable but very different on the other variable. This runs the risk of selecting subjects who are really different on both variables because extreme scores are less reliable and are more likely to regress to the mean. In the present study, we dealt with this problem by selecting subjects on the basis of two reading comprehension and two spelling test scores rather than just one reading and spelling score. Also we obtained confirmation from other tasks we gave that our subjects did not differ on language measures other than spelling. Thus, our study does not appear to be flawed by the problem of regression to the mean.

Although dysgraphics and normals were equivalent in reading comprehension and vocabulary learning in the present study, we found that they were not equivalent on the CTBS math subtest. Dysgraphic spellers received lower scores than normal spellers, $M = 66.4$ vs. 76.3 percentile, $F(1, 64) = 6.107$, $p < 0.05$. Perhaps similar factors account for math and spelling weaknesses, for example, analytic learning style, or attention to details, or propensity to learn rules (Morrison, 1984). These possibilities await study.

To summarize, we believe we have shown that dysgraphics spell words by eye as well as by ear rather than just by ear, at least in some circumstances. In this respect, they do not differ from normal spellers in using information gained by reading words to spell them. The primary way that they differ from normal spellers is in their ability to remember complete spellings of words when they read them. Normal spellers have better phonological recoding skill, and they possess knowledge about how English spellings are structured beyond the phoneme—grapheme level. This enables them to process letters in the spellings of words more completely when they read the words, to retain these spellings more completely in memory to spell the words, and to generate better guesses about unknown word spellings. Dysgraphics have knowledge about phoneme—grapheme relations that they can use to store phonetically interpretable letters in memory and to generate phonetically plausible spellings. However, they are not as skilled at phonological recording and they lack higher level knowledge of the orthographic system. This weakens their ability to process the phonemic function of letters as well as higher level patterns when they read words and to generate plausible spelling patterns beyond the phonetic level.

NOTES

[1] By phonetic spelling strategy we mean a sequential analytic approach in which rules are used to select letters or digraphs to symbolize systematically the sequence of sounds detected in pronunciations. We have assumed that the letter selection process used by dysgraphics does not include hierarchical conditional rules in which silent marker letters determine the sounds of preceding letters, for example, final E lengthening a preceding vowel, and double consonants shortening a preceding vowel (Marsh *et al.,* 1981; Venezky, 1970). Such conditional rules applied to the set of target words used here would account for silent letters in two words, Frosin*one* and Apenn*ines*, and double letters in two words, inc*ess*antly and C*omm*odus. Even if dysgraphics knew and used these rules, this would still not account fully for the extent of their correct production of silent and double letters in the present study.

[2] The basic spelling rules that we adopted were: long vowels spelled with letters having those sounds in their names (A, E, I, O, U); short vowels spelled A for /ă/, E for /ĕ/, I for /ĭ/, o for /ŏ/, U for /ŭ/; standard spellings of /l/, /g/, /f/, /r/, /n/, /t/, /v/, /p/, /m/, /b/, /h/, /d/; SH for /š/; CH for /č/; Y for final /ē/; QU for initial /kw/; S for /z/; C for /k/; U for schwa.

REFERENCES

Becker, W. C., Dixon, R. and Anderson-Inman, L.: 1980, *Morphographic and Root Word Analysis of 26,000 High Frequency Words*, University of Oregon College of Education, Eugene, Oregon.

Cronnell, B.: 1978, 'Phonics for reading vs. phonics for spelling', *Reading Teacher* **32**, 337—340.

Drake, D. A. and Ehri, L. C.: 1984, 'Spelling acquisition: Effects of pronouncing words on memory for their spellings', *Cognition and Instruction* **1**, 297—320.

Ehri, L. C.: 1980, 'The development of orthographic images', in U. Frith (ed.), *Cognitive Processes in Spelling*, pp. 311—338, Academic Press, London.

Ehri, L. C.: 1984, 'How orthography alters spoken language competencies in children learning to read and spell', in J. Downing and R. Valtin (eds.), *Language Awareness and Learning to Read*, pp. 119—147, Springer Verlag, New York.

Ehri, L. C.: 1986, 'Sources of difficulty in learning to spell and read', in M. L. Wolraich and D. Routh (eds.), *Advances in Developmental and Behavioral Pediatrics*, Vol. 7, pp. 121—195, JAI Press, Greenwich, Conn.

Ehri L. C.: 1987, 'Learning to read and spell words', *Journal of Reading Behavior* **19**, 5—31.

Ehri, L. C. (in press), 'Reconceptualizing the development of sight word reading and its relationship to recoding', in P. Gough, L. Ehri and Treiman (eds.), *Reading Acquisition*, Erlbaum, Hillsdale, NJ.

Ehri, L. C. and Roberts, K. T.: 1979, 'Do beginners learn printed words better in contexts or in isolation?', *Child Development* **50**, 675—685.

Ehri, L. C. and Wilce, L. S.: 1979, 'The mnemonic value of orthography among beginning readers', *Journal of Educational Psychology* **71**, 26—40.

Ehri, L. C. and Wilce, L. S.: 1980a, 'Do beginners learn to read function words better in sentences or in lists?', *Reading Research Quarterly* **15**, 451—476.

Ehri, L. C. and Wilce, L. S.: 1980b, 'The influence of orthography on readers' conceptualization of the phonemic structure of words', *Applied Psycholinguistics* **1**, 371—385.

Ehri, L. C. and Wilce, L. S.: 1982, 'The salience of silent letters in children's memory for word spellings', *Memory and Cognition* **10**, 155—166.

Ehri, L. C. and Wilce, L. C.: 1986, 'The influence of spellings on speech: Are alveolar flaps /d/ or /t/?', in D. Yaden and S. Templeton (eds.), *Metalinguistic Awareness and Beginning Literacy*, pp. 101—114, Heinemann Educational Books, Exeter, NH.

Frith, U.: 1978, 'From print to meaning and from print to sound, or how to read without knowing how to spell', *Visible Language* **12**, 43—54.

Frith, U.: 1979, 'Reading by eye and writing by ear', in P. A. Kolers, M. Wrolstad and H. Bouma (eds.), *Processing of Visible Language*, Vol. 1, pp. 379—390, Plenum Press, New York.

Frith, U.: 1980, 'Unexpected spelling problems', in U. Frith (ed.), *Cognitive Processes in Spelling*, pp. 495—515, Academic Press, London.

Hanna, P. R., Hanna, J. S., Hodges, R. E. and Rudorf, E. H.: 1966, *Phoneme—grapheme Correspondences as Cues to Spelling Improvement*, U.S. Government Printing Office, Washington, D.C.

Liberman, A. M., Cooper, F. S., Shankweiler, D. P., and Studdert-Kennedy, M.: 1967, 'Perception of the speech code', *Psychological Review* **74**, 431—461.

Marsh, G., Friedman, M., Welch, V. and Desberg, P.: 1980, 'The development of strategies in spelling', in U. Frith (ed.), *Cognitive Processes in Spelling*, pp. 339—353, Academic Press, London.

Marsh, G., Friedman, M., Welch, V. and Desberg, P.: 1981, 'A cognitive-developmental theory of reading acquisition', in G. E. Mackinnon and T. G. Waller (eds.), *Reading Research: Advances in Theory and Practice*, Vol. 3, pp. 199—221, Academic Press, New York.

Morrison, F. J.: 1984, 'Reading disability: A problem in rule learning and word decoding', *Developmental Review* **4**, 36—47.

Shanahan, T.: 1984, 'Nature of the reading-writing relation: An exploratory multivariate analysis', *Journal of Educational Psychology* **76**, 446—477.

Simon, D. P.: 1976, 'Spelling: A task analysis', *Instructional Science* **5**, 277—302.

Simon, D. P. and Simon, H. A.: 1973, 'Alternative uses of phonemic information in spelling', *Review of Educational Research* **43**, 115—137.

Stanovich, K. E.: 1980, 'Toward an interactive-compensatory model of individual differences in the development of reading fluency', *Reading Research Quarterly* **16**, 32—71.

Stanovich, K. E.: 1986, 'Matthew effects in reading: Some consequences of individual differences in the acquisition of literacy', *Reading Research Quarterly* **21**, 360—407.

Venezky, R. L.: 1970, *The Structure of English Orthography*, Mouton, The Hague.

APPENDIX

Story Read by Subjects in the Silent Context Condition

Caligula, the Emperor of Rome from 37 to 41 A.D., owned what may have been history's most pampered horse. (Caligula, He) loved and cared for this special horse, whose name was Incitatus, in a most unusual way.

(Incitatus, The horse) lived at Frosinone, a palace at the base of Mt. Vesuvius in the Apennines mountain range in Italy. The seismic activity of this active volcano was believed to give the royal occupants of the palace divine powers.

At (Frosinone, the palace) (Incitatus, the horse) was surrounded by the splendor and riches of royalty. His crystalline stall had an ivory manger at a golden water bowl. An average citizen of Rome had far fewer comforts. The horse ate better quality food than most of the people of his day. Slaves attended (Incitatus, the horse) incessantly while musicians entertained him with gentle cantatas.

Each evening (Incitatus, the horse) had dinner in a large banquet hall with senators and other important guests. The perfumed horse wore elegant jeweled collars to these feasts. What happened if an invited guest did not care to dine with a horse? Such an uncooperative person could face banishment.

(Caligula, The emperor) gave his horse virtually every luxury. He even tried to appoint (Incitatus, the horse) to the office of Consullar, a post once held by Julius Caesar. The horse did not, however, assume office. A palace guard, Commodus, felt that (Caligula, the emperor) had carried his bizarre affection for an equinal friend to excess and murdered the emperor to end his horrendous rule. History did not record the precise fate of (Incitatus, the horse).

HYLA RUBIN

MORPHOLOGICAL KNOWLEDGE AND WRITING ABILITY

The development of morphological knowledge and its relationship to writing ability will be examined in this chapter. Such an examination is warranted because, in spelling, the child needs to understand the internal structure of words. Specifically, the child needs to understand that words have a morphophonemic structure, that is, that phonemic elements combine to form morphemes, which combine to form inflected and derived versions of words. Previous work has suggested that although an implicit understanding of the morphophonemic structure of words may be sufficient for spoken language proficiency, written language proficiency demands both an implicit *and* an explicit understanding of morphophonemic structure (Liberman, 1971, 1973, 1983; Liberman, *et al.*, 1974; Mattingly, 1972).

Accordingly, research on two aspects of morphological knowledge, implicit and explicit, will be reviewed in relation to writing ability. The first, implicit knowledge, refers to a tacit understanding of the morphological rule system of the language. It has been assessed by measuring children's ability to apply morphological rules to nonsense base words in an elicited spoken language task. The second, explicit morphological knowledge, or awareness of the morphophonemic structure of the language, refers to the *explicit* understanding that phonemes form morphemes and that morphemes form inflected and derived versions of words. Explicit morphological knowledge has been assessed by testing children's ability to identify base morphemes in inflected forms of words. Writing ability has only recently been examined in relation to either of these aspects of morphological knowledge. Following the presentation of selected results from three current studies, implications and procedures for educational assessment and programming will be discussed.

1. WRITING AND LEVELS OF MORPHOLOGICAL KNOWLEDGE

Results of studies of spelling and written expression to date invite us to inquire into the relationship of morphological knowledge and writing ability, since inflected and derived forms of words have been found to pose difficulties both for beginning spellers and for children and adults with learning problems. For example, studies of spelling ability of college students indicate that poor spellers fail most dramatically on those words that require sensitivity to morphophonemic structure (Fischer, 1980; Hanson, *et al.*, 1983). In addition, clinicians frequently report that child-

R. M. Joshi (ed.), Written Language Disorders, 43–69.
© 1991 *Kluwer Academic Publishers. Printed in the Netherlands.*

ren's errors in spelling (and in reading) include the omission and substitution of inflectional markers and substitution of base words for derived
words or one derived form of a word for another (Cicci, 1980). Although
it has been demonstrated that children and adults with learning problems
make more of these errors when writing than do other children and adults
(Anderson, 1982; Liberman, *et al.*, 1985; Moran, 1981; Myklebust,
1973), possible reasons for the occurrence of these errors have not been
addressed.

The basis for such errors when writing might fall into one of two
categories. On the one hand, they might represent part of a general
tendency to misspell words. If this is the case, omissions of inflectional
endings, for example, might be but one instance of a more pervasive
pattern of final consonant omissions. On the other hand, they might
reflect an underlying deficit in morphological knowledge. If that is the
case, it should be possible to expose this deficit at other levels and
demonstrate that children and adults who make such errors in their
written language also perform poorly in their attempts to use morphological rules in spoken language (implicit knowledge) or to analyze the
internal morphemic structure of words (explicit knowledge).

Although the relationship between morphological knowledge and writing ability has not been examined directly, there is good reason to
anticipate that children who make morphemic errors when writing are
indeed deficient in their underlying morphological skills. Several studies
have demonstrated that children with reading problems have difficulty
applying morphological rules to new words (Brittain, 1970; Doehring,
et al., 1981; Vogel, 1975, 1983; Wiig, *et al.*, 1973). In all of these studies,
morphological knowledge has been assessed by an elicited spoken language
task that requires the application of basic inflectional and derivational
rules of morphology to nonsense base words (Berko, 1958; Berry and
Talbott, 1966). This method is used in order to determine that children
are actually applying the morphological rules that they have mastered and
are not just producing memorized vocabulary items. It has been found that
normally developing children master these rules between the ages of four
and seven (Brown, 1973; deVilliers and deVilliers, 1973; Selby, 1972;
Templin, 1957). In contrast, children with learning problems develop this
type of morphological knowledge more slowly, although they are found to
follow the same sequence in their rule acquisition.

Research has not yet examined whether morpheme use is directly
related to linguistic skills other than reading, or why these relationships
might exist. But given the evidence above, one might expect there to be a
strong relationship between the ability to use morphemes correctly in
spoken language and in written language since, in both cases, this ability
would depend on the acquisition of morphological rules and access to
them in the lexicon. However, while the implicit understanding of mor-

phophonemic structure should be the minimum requirement for morpheme use in writing, the further stage of *explicit* understanding of the morphophonemic structure of English would be expected to differentiate clearly between proficient and poorer writers.

2. EXPLICIT AWARENESS OF PHONEMIC STRUCTURE

Previous research studies have demonstrated that the ability to explicitly analyze the internal structure of words is a critical component in learning to read (Blachman, 1983; Fox and Routh, 1980; Liberman, *et al.*, 1974; Lundberg, *et al.*, 1980; Treiman and Baron, 1981) and in learning to spell (Perin, 1983; Liberman *et al.*, 1985; Zifcak, 1981). In the reading studies, the ability to analyze spoken words into syllabic and phonemic segments has been found to be highly related to letter naming and word recognition performance in kindergarten, first and second grade children. In the spelling studies, phonemic segmentation ability has been found to be significantly related to dictated spelling performance in kindergarteners (Liberman *et al.*, 1985), first graders (Zifcak, 1981) and adolescents (Perin, 1983).

Research into the structural analysis of spoken words and its relationship to reading and writing abilities has yielded valuable theoretical and instructional information thus far. It is clear that children with reading and spelling problems are less able than their normally achieving peers to analyze spoken words into their constituent phonemes. However, many questions about this relationship remain unanswered. It is of particular concern that the ability to analyze spoken words into their constituent morphemes has received so little attention. Since the English orthography, like the spoken language it represents, is morphophonemic (Chomsky and Halle, 1968; Liberman, *et al.*, 1980), a critical step in its mastery should be the ability to analyze the internal structure of a word as a function of both its morphemic and phonemic structure.

3. EXPLICIT KNOWLEDGE OF MORPHOPHONEMIC STRUCTURE

Recent studies have begun to examine the explicit understanding of morphophonemic structure in children. Derwing and Baker (1977, 1979) have investigated the development of morpheme identification ability in children in grades 3 through college. They provided their subjects with word pairs which were varied for semantic and phonetic similarity, such as *teach-teacher, slip-slipper, cup-cupboard,* and *moon-month.* The subjects were required to read each pair and indicate if one word "came from the other", using a 5-point scale to specify the degree of relatedness. Performance correlated with age and degree of semantic and phonetic relationship between the paired words. The authors concluded that morpheme recognition ability may develop as much through instructional experience as through language acquisition and suggested that it would be difficult to sort out the contributions of these two sources of linguistic knowledge.

Although this research into the explicit analysis of morphemic structure is provocative, similar studies have not been conducted with children who demonstrate learning problems or with children below third grade. It would be expected that if younger children were deficient in their ability to use morphemes in spoken language, which would reflect their implicit awareness of morphological structure, they would also be deficient in their ability to recognize base morphemes within two-morpheme words, or their explicit awareness of morphological structure. If these abilities were found to be related to each other and to morpheme use in early spelling, it would be possible to demonstrate the necessity of helping young children develop sensitivity to morphemic structure through direct instruction. An examination of these abilites in young children would also serve to establish levels of morphological knowledge that can normally be expected, in order to more profitably study the relationship of writing to morphological knowledge in individuals who experience written language difficulties.

4. CURRENT STUDIES OF MORPHOLOGICAL KNOWLEDGE AND SPELLING ABILITY

The research discussed below was designed to examine the relationship between implicit knowledge of morphemic structure, as measured by the ability to apply morphological rules to new words, and explicit knowledge of morphemic structure, as measured by the ability to identify base words within two-morpheme words. Furthermore, the relationship between performance on these spoken language tasks and the ability to represent base morphemes and inflectional morphemes in writing was investigated, using a variety of tasks judged to be appropriate for the different age levels included in these studies.

STUDY 1: *Morphological Knowledge and Beginning Spelling Ability* (Rubin, 1984, 1987)

Subjects

The subjects were children selected from kindergarten and first-grade classes in a suburban Connecticut public school. The available 128 children (59 kindergarteners and 69 first graders) demonstrated adequate vision and hearing and were judged to have normal intelligence by their classroom teachers and the school psychologist. All were monolingual speakers of General American English dialect. During a one-week period, they were individually given the *Berry—Talbott Language Test* (Berry and Talbott, 1966), a measure of elicited morpheme production in spoken language. This test required them to apply basic inflectional and derivational rules of morphology to nonsense base words by completing spoken sentences when shown illustrative pictures. For example,

> "This is a nad who knows how to trom. He is tromming. He did the same thing yesterday. What did he do yesterday? Yesterday he ___."

The accompanying picture is presented in Figure 1.

Four groups were formed by selecting those children from each grade who scored within the highest and lowest thirds of the distribution of scores on the *Berry—Talbott Language Test*. The children from the highest third of the kindergarten and first-grade distributions will be referred to as the high kindergarteners and high first graders. Similarly, the subjects from the lowest third of the kindergarten and first-grade distributions will be referred to as the low kindergarteners and low first graders. The mean age and test scores for each group are summarized in Table 1. All four groups differed significantly from each other in their performance on the *Berry—Talbott*.

Materials and Specific Procedures

The 86 children in the four groups were tested further to determine the relationship of their morpheme use in spoken language to their morpheme

TABLE 1

Berry—Talbott Language Test: Grouped mean scores (and standard deviations) for kindergarteners and first graders

	Kindergarteners		First Graders	
	Low	High	Low	High
n	21	19	22	24
Berry—Talbott	10.8	24.7	14.1	28.0
	(3.3)	(2.5)	(4.1)	(3.3)
Age (years—months)	5—5	5—5	6—5	6—5

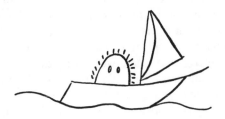

Fig. 1. Sample item: *Berry—Talbott Language Test*.

use in writing and to their explicit morpheme analysis ability. During the one-week period following administraation of the *Berry—Talbott Language Test* (1966), each of the four groups of children was given a dictated experimental spelling test in a half-hour group session. This measure was designed to assess the children's representation of base and inflectional morphemes in the early stages of their experience with written language. Although previous studies that document morphemic errors in writing had analyzed spontaneous writing samples, it was not considered reasonable to elicit writing samples in the present study since the children tested were only in the fifth month of kindergarten and first grade. However, it was important to study children of this age, as it was expected that they would demonstrate sufficient variability in their levels of implicit and explicit knowledge of morphological structure of spoken words to enable us to learn more about the course of this development. Furthermore, previous studies of invented spelling (Read, 1971, 1975) have demonstrated that by age 5 many children are able to analyze words into their constituent phonemes and use their knowledge of letter names to "invent" written representations of the spoken words. By scoring for the number of morphemes represented in writing rather than for correctness of spelling, it seemed reasonable to use a dictated spelling task as an early indication of the ability to represent inflectional morphemes in written form. In this way, both spoken and written language measures of the morphological knowledge of young children could be obtained.

The experimental spelling test contained 31 words that were considered to be part of the average kindergartener's spoken vocabulary. Twenty-one words were organized according to morphemic structure (one or two morphemes) and type of final consonant cluster (nasal or non-nasal). Three experimental words were given in each of the following categories: (1) two-morpheme words ending in *md* (*hummed, jammed, dimmed*), (2) one-morpheme words ending in *nd* (*wind, band, kind*), (3) two-morpheme words ending in *nd* (*pinned, canned, lined*), (4) one-morpheme words ending in *nt* (*tent, pant, hint*), (5) two-morpheme words ending in *nt* (*bent, can't, don't*), (6) one-morpheme words ending in *st* (*list, dust, nest*), and (7) two-morpheme words ending in *st* (*kissed, fussed, messed*). Ten words were used as fillers to reduce the possible priming effects of the experimental words. Five of the fillers were one-morpheme words (*winter, candy, dinner, money*, and *wise*) and five were two-morpheme words (*hunter, windy, winner, funny*, and *pies*). The experimental and filler words were randomized and each word was dictated, then used in a meaningful sentence and repeated. To insure consistent presentation of the stimuli, the word and sentence script was recorded by a speaker of General American English and was presented on tape. The children were instructed to write each word on a pre-numbered response form.

During the following three-week period, each child was given the experimental measures of morpheme analysis and a letter-naming task in an individual testing session of approximately 20 minutes.

The experimental morpheme analysis task was designed to assess the ability to analyze a spoken word into its constituent morphemes by requiring each child to identify base morphemes within words. This task consisted of the same 31 words that were used for spelling. The child was asked questions such as "Is there a smaller word in *list* that means something like *list*?" or "Is there a smaller word in *kissed* that means something like *kissed*?" for each of the words. For one-morpheme words (such as *list, pant,* and *wind*), the child was supposed to respond "No". For two-morpheme words (such as *kissed, can't,* and *pinned*), the child was supposed to respond "Yes" and supply the base word.

These procedures were demonstrated in six training trials in the following manner. First, the child listened to each question and responded spontaneously. If the response was incorrect, the examiner repeated the question, provided the correct response along with a brief explanation, and asked the question again. This procedure was repeated once if needed. Words that contained smaller words that were not related to the stimulus word (such as *pillow* and *sink*) were included in the training trials and required "no" responses. On the test trials, no demonstrations or feedback were given.

Results

Implicit Morphological Knowledge and Spelling Ability. Letter-naming scores were tabulated and showed that all but the low kindergarten children could name over 90% of the letters of the alphabet.

For each child, the percentage of written words with final consonant omissions was also tabulated. Any response in which the final consonant was omitted was counted here, whether the remainder of the word was spelled accurately or not. That is, for the word *canned*, responses such as *canned, kand, cnd,* and *knd* were considered complete representations, but responses such as *can, kan, cn,* and *kn* were coded as final consonant omissions. (The words were also scored for other types of errors that are beyond the scope of this discussion. It is important to realize, therefore, that the remaining percentage of words for each group did not consist of correctly spelled words. In fact, words were *never* scored for accuracy of spelling, but rather for completeness of representation of base and inflectional morphemes.) The high first graders omitted final consonants from 3% of the words, the high kindergarteners from 10%, the low first graders from 17%, and the low kindergarteners from 10%. (Since low kindergarteners were not able to name the letters of the alphabet, a skill needed for invented spelling, their spelling results will not be discussed further here.) The results suggest that the ability to represent final consonants in written language is significantly related to morphological knowledge in spoken language and is not significantly related to grade level independent of linguistic ability. This is seen by the fact that low first graders omitted more final consonants than did either the high first graders or the high kindergarteners. Furthermore, when the data are examined as a function of both morphemic and phonemic structure, they indicate that, in omitting final consonants in their spelling, children tend not to be influenced by the phonemic structure of the words. It was found that the percentage of error on words ending in nasal and non-nasal consonant clusters was roughly the same — 8% and 7% respectively. In contrast, there was a striking effect of morphemic structure. Whereas children omitted final consonants from only 4% of one-morpheme words, they omitted final consonants from 11% of two-morpheme words, a difference which was highly significant. It is clear from these results that final consonants were omitted more often from two-morpheme than from one-morpheme words, and that it was the morphologically less knowledgeable first graders who were omitting those inflectional morphemes.

Implicit and Explicit Levels of Morphological Knowledge. In the morpheme analysis task, a two-morpheme word (such as *pinned*) was scored as correct if the child (1) responded "Yes" and supplied the correct base form of the word (*pin*), and (2) responded "No" to a phonemically similar one-morpheme word (*wind*). (The *md* words [*hummed, jammed, dimmed*] were excluded from this scoring system because there are no one-morpheme words in English that end in *md*.) The two-pronged scoring system was necessary to counter possible effects of response bias. Without such a system, indiscriminate "no" responses would result in higher scores than indiscriminate "yes" responses, since "yes" responses had to be accompanied by the correct base word and "no" responses had no such control.

Using this scoring system, the percentage of correctly analyzed word pairs was tabulated for each child. Both high first graders and high kindergarteners analyzed 48% of the pairs correctly, low first graders 24%, and low kindergarteners 3%. The correlation between the number of pairs a child analyzed correctly and morpheme use in spoken language proved to be significant, ($r[84] = 0.63$, $p < 0.001$), indicating a strong relationship between implicit and explicit levels of morphological knowledge.

What is particularly notable about these results is that children with high levels of implicit morphological knowledge in the elicited spoken language task performed equally well on the explicit analysis task regardless of grade level differences. Therefore, the ability to analyze morphemic structure explicitly, at least as measured by this task and at this point in development, seems to be more highly related to implicit morphological knowledge in spoken language than to grade level factors such as age and amount of instructional experience.

Considering previous research on phonemic analysis, it was enlightening to examine the types of errors made by the low kindergarteners and low first graders when they attempted to analyze the morphemic structure of spoken words explicitly. It was found that many of these children could manipulate phonemic segments without understanding morphemic structure. For example, in response to the questions "Is there a smaller word in *kind* that means something like *kind*?" and "Is there a smaller word in *dust* that means something like *dust*?", they often responded "Yes, *kin*" or "Yes, *tind*" or "Yes, *dus*" or "Yes, *tust*". This finding highlights the importance of examining the ability to analyze explicitly the morphemic, as well as the phonemic, structure of words.

STUDY 2: *Morphological Knowledge and Writing Ability; a Follow-up of the Kindergarten and First Grade Children* (Rubin, 1985)

Subjects

The subjects in this study were 72 of the 86 children who participated in the previous study. They will now be referred to as high and low first and second graders.

Materials and Specific Procedures

During a one-week period at the end of the school year (one and one-half years after the original testing), each of the four groups of children was given three writing tasks in three group testing sessions of 30 minutes. Since their spelling performance had previously been measured at the single word level only, these further measures were designed to assess their ability to represent inflectional morphemes in more demanding writing tasks. The tasks were administered one day apart in the following order:

(1) Spontaneous writing samples were collected, using a transparency of one of the stimulus pictures from the "I Wonder" cards (#W-9) in the Peabody Language Development Kit, Level 2 (Dunn and Smith, 1965). The picture was shown on a screen to each group of children, who were given one-half hour to write a spontaneous description of it. They were instructed to look at the picture and write a story about it after taking a few minutes to think. Samples were scored for inclusion and substitution of inflectional morphemes.

(2) Elicited writing samples were collected, using 10 transparencies of two line-drawings each. Each pair of drawings contrasted an action in progress (in the first drawing) with the same action completed (in the second). This contrast was used to elicit the regular past tense morpheme by instructing the children to write a description of the second picture. They were given two training trials to ensure comprehension of the task. Sentences were scored for inclusion of inflectional past tense morphemes.

(3) Sentences were dictated to the children, who were instructed to write each one after hearing it twice. Each sentence contained one of the 31 words used in the single-word dictated spelling task in Study 1. To insure consistent presentation of the stimuli, all of the sentences were recorded by a speaker of General American English and presented on tape. Sentences were scored for inclusion of final consonants on one- and two-morpheme words.

Results

Prior to presenting the results of the follow-up testing, it is relevant to mention the type of instructional program that had been used during the school year. For all of the children in the primary grades, a spelling program emphasizing structural analysis of orthographically regular base words and inflectional endings (Szolusha, *et al.*, 1984) had been implemented on a daily basis in the classrooms. It was of particular interest, considering this change in teaching methodology, to see if any of the children would still demonstrate morphemic errors in their writing.

Overall, the results yielded a much lower incidence of morphemic errors, in all writing tasks, than was anticipated based on previous research findings (Anderson, 1982; Liberman *et al.*, 1985; Moran, 1981; Myklebust, 1973) and clinical observations (Cicci, 1980). To begin with, neither the high second graders, high first graders, nor low second graders omitted final consonants from one-morpheme or two-morpheme words in the dictated sentence task. The low first graders, however, omitted final consonants from 8% of the one-morpheme words and from 15% of the two-morpheme words when writing to dictation. On the elicited writing task, where all 10 target words required past tense inflectional morphemes, the same pattern emerged: final consonants were not usually omitted by the high second graders, high first graders, or low second graders. However, the low first graders omitted inflectional morphemes from 17% of the target words. Examples of elicited writing responses are presented in Appendix 1. Finally, when writing spontaneously, children in the two low groups made three times as many morphemic errors as children in the two high groups, although the frequency of this type of error never exceeded 10% of the total errors. Samples of spontaneous writing are presented in Appendix 2.

Although a higher percentage of morphemic errors in writing was anticipated than was obtained, especially in the spontaneous writing condition, there are several factors to consider when interpreting the obtained results. First of all, it is difficult to ensure that young children will generate enough output to allow an investigator to describe accurately their ability (or inability) to use inflected forms of words correctly when writing spontaneously. (Nonetheless, children in the low first- and second-grade groups did demonstrate higher ratios of morphemic errors to total errors in their spontaneous samples than children in the high groups.) The difficulties inherent in collecting representative spontaneous writing samples reinforce the need to evaluate writing performance across more than one task (Gregg, 1983). In this respect, elicited writing tasks may be an important measure to be used in conjunction with more spontaneous tasks. Furthermore, if elicited and dictated sentence-writing results continue to yield similar results, then dictated tasks may be an even more efficient means of collecting data. Ongoing research is attempting to determine which measures of written output are most valid.

The incidence of morphemic errors in writing could also have been affected by the type of spelling instruction being given during the school year prior to the follow-up testing. Since this instruction emphasized analysis of the internal structure of orthographically regular words and was used on a daily basis in the first- and second-grade classrooms, it is possible that the low incidence of morphemic errors may be (at least partially) attributable to its success.

Nonetheless, the low first graders omitted a considerable number of inflectional morphemes in both the elicited and dictated writing tasks, and in the dictated task, omitted final consonants from two-morpheme words twice as frequently as from one-morpheme words.

The possibility also exists that the children who demonstrated low levels of morphological knowledge in the middle of first grade had developed adequate linguistic skills by the end of second grade. Unfortunately, neither the implicit nor explicit levels of morphological knowledge were measured again in the children participating in the follow-up testing. Since neither level was found to have developed fully by first grade, and since morphemic errors in writing persist in some older children and adults, it is important to continue to examine the course of development of morphological knowledge.

STUDY 3: *Morphological Knowledge and Writing Ability in Second Graders and in Adult Poor Readers* (Rubin and Patterson, and Kantor, in press)

Subjects

The three groups of subjects comprised (1) ten normally achieving second-grade children in a suburban Ontario public school system, (2) ten second graders in the same school system, designated as language-disabled on a standardized test battery given by a certified speech-language pathologist, and (3) seven adults who attended an Ontario remedial reading center. All subjects were monolingual speakers of English and demonstrated adequate vision and hearing. The normally achieving second-grade subjects were judged to have normal intelligence by their classroom teacher and/or the school psychologist; all other subjects demonstrated normal functioning on standardized intelligence tests.

Materials and Specific Procedures

During a five-week period, each of the subjects attended two testing sessions. In the first, an individual session of 30 minutes, the *Berry—Talbott Language Test* and an expanded version of the morpheme analysis task used in Study 1 were given. In the second, a group session of 40 minutes, two writing tasks that were used in Study 2 were administered: (1) the dictated sentence writing task (however, only the 21 words that ended in consonant clusters were used this time), and (2) the spontaneous writing task.

The morpheme analysis task used in Study 1 was expanded to examine the effect of two-syllable words more closely. The original task (Rubin, 1984) included ten pairs of one-syllable words and only four pairs of two-syllable words. When the data were analyzed to determine if subjects were better able to identify base words within two-morpheme words when the base morpheme was a separate syllable than when it was not, no significant effect was obtained. It was felt that a syllabic effect may not have been obtained because there were so few pairs of two-syllable words. Therefore, a second stimulus list was developed for the present study, consisting of six pairs of one-syllable words and 14 pairs of multisyllable words. Procedures for task administration were the same as in Study 1. The results discussed below refer to calculations done on the two combined stimulus lists, i.e. a total of 16 one-syllable word pairs and 18 two-syllable word pairs.

Results

Implicit Morphological Knowledge. For each subject, the number of correctly inflected words on the *Berry—Talbott Language Test* was tabulated. Of 38 items, the normally achieving second graders and adult poor readers correctly inflected a mean of 23 words, and the language-disabled second graders 11. Although the second-grade experimental group performed significantly more poorly than either of the other two groups, neither the second-grade control group nor the adult poor readers correctly inflected more than 65% of the items. These results demonstrate that normally achieving second graders are still acquiring implicit morphological knowledge and that adult poor readers perform at the same level as the second-grade control subjects, in spite of maturation and many more years of exposure to spoken and written language.

Explicit Morphological Knowledge. Scoring procedures for the expanded morpheme analysis task paralleled those used in Study 1 for the original task. The pattern of results is strikingly similar to that obtained for implicit morphological knowledge, as the language-disabled second graders performed significantly more poorly (30% of the pairs were analyzed correctly) than either of the other two groups, both of whom performed very similarly (63%). Again, although out-performing the language-disabled second graders, neither of the other groups of subjects had mastered the ability to analyze the internal morphemic structure of spoken words, indicating that explicit morphological knowledge was still being acquired by normally achieving second graders and that adult poor readers had not developed this skill as a result of instructional experience or maturation.

In an effort to identify factors that might affect the difficulty of this task, the data were analyzed as a function of the syllabic structure of the word pairs. This was done to determine if subjects would be more successful at identifying base words in two-morpheme words that were bisyllabic, since the morphemic and syllabic boundaries of these words would coincide, than in single-syllable two-morpheme words. It was found that language-disabled second graders and adult poor readers performed significantly better when analyzing pairs of two-syllable words than pairs of one-syllable words (language-disabled second graders, 40% versus 22%; adult poor readers, 76% versus 50%), although the normally achieving second graders performed similarly in the two conditions (69% versus 61%). These results suggest that the experimental groups are at a more serious disadvantage than the control group when faced with the task of analyzing the morphemic structure of one-syllable words, perhaps because recognition of the base and inflectional morphemes is not facilitated by the syllabic structure of the words.

Morpheme Use in Writing. On the dictated sentence-writing task, the percentage of one- and two-morpheme words with final consonant omissions was calculated for each subject. Normally achieving second graders omitted very few final consonants for either word type (2% for one-morpheme words, 6% for two-morpheme words), and adult poor readers omitted an equal number of final consonants for each word type (16%). Only the language-disabled second graders omitted significantly more final consonants when writing two-morpheme (39%) than one-morpheme (24%) words. The fact that language-disabled children demonstrated particular difficulty using final consonants that functioned as inflectional morphemes supports previous dictated spelling results with children who lacked a high level of morphological knowledge (Rubin, 1984). The finding that adult poor readers did not show particular difficulty with morpheme use in this task raises two possibilities. First of all, this dictated sentence-writing task may not have been very demanding for them. Secondly, this group of adults might not show morphemic errors in writing under any conditions.

Turning to the spontaneous writing results, two tabulations were made for each subject: total errors, and the percentage of these errors that were morphemic in nature. Of their total errors, normally developing second graders made morphemic errors 2% of the time, language disabled children 12% and adults 13%. Both of the experimental groups differed significantly from the second grade control subjects on this task. An example of spontaneous writing of an adult subject is presented in Appendix 3.

5. GENERAL DISCUSSION

The purpose of these studies was to investigate the development of morphological knowledge and its relationship to writing ability in young children and in adults with reading problems. Two levels of morphological knowledge were examined, since previous research had suggested that one needs to understand morphophonemic structure both implicitly and explicitly in order to spell. Although previous studies had concluded that written language proficiency requires an explicit understanding of morphophonemic structure, the ability of young children and adult poor readers to analyze the internal structure of words had been examined at the phonemic but not at the morphemic level of language.

It was found, in accordance with previous studies of language acquisition, that children in kindergarten, first and second grades are still developing implicit morphological knowledge (as measured by the *Berry—Talbott*), and that they use certain morphological rules before others. Unfortunately, it was also found that adult poor readers performed only as well as normally achieving second graders, who had far from mastered the implicit morphological knowledge task. Notably, in view of the large number of past tense items in the stimuli that were used to assess writing and explicit analysis abilities, most of the subjects in these studies successfully applied the morphological rules for regular past tense (in the nonsense words *trommed, flitched, linged,* and *bazinged*).

In addition, it was found that implicit morphological knowledge does not develop solely as a function of factors associated with maturation and amount of instructional experience. This was demonstrated, in the first study, by the fact that some kindergarteners (the high group) performed significantly better than some first graders (the low group) and, in the third study, by the poor performance of the adults, whose results paralleled those of previously studied adult poor readers (Liberman *et al.*, 1985). However, the role of factors associated with instructional experience should not be disregarded, since, in the first study, high first graders performed significantly better than high kindergarteners, and low first graders performed significantly better than low kindergarteners. What is clear is that the subjects in these studies vary greatly in their implicit knowledge of the morphology and that this variability affects their writing ability.

In fact, implicit morphological knowledge had a more significant effect than amount of instructional experience on the tendency of these subjects to omit inflectional morphemes in writing. This was seen, in the first study, by the fact that low first graders made relatively more of these errors than either high first graders or high kindergarteners, and, in the third study, by the significant differences obtained between the language-disabled and normally achieving second graders on both writing tasks, as well as by the adults' errors when writing spontaneously. However, results of the follow-up study suggest that morpheme use in writing may in fact be affected by instructional experience when that instruction includes a specific focus on analysis of the internal morphemic structure of words. When studied one year later, the second graders who were previously in the low first grade group appear to have benefited greatly from regular classroom instruction in structural analysis. On the other hand, adult poor readers, in the third study and in previous work (Liberman *et al.*, 1985), demonstrate persistent morphemic errors in writing, in spite of years of reportedly traditional forms of written language instruction. Of course, direct comparisons cannot be made between these different populations, but the results do support the position that instructional programming should address the morphophonemic aspects of learning to spell (and to read).

The results of the morphemic analysis task used in these studies also support the need to help subjects such as ours to develop the sensitivity to morphophonemic structure that they need to become proficient language users. To begin with, explicit morphological knowledge, at least as measured by the identification task used in these studies, was found consistently to be highly related to both implicit morphological knowledge and to morpheme use in writing. Secondly, the ability to analyze the morphophonemic structure of a word was found to be independent of instructional experience to some degree for both young children and adult poor readers, since high kindergarteners performed significantly better than low first graders, and since adult poor readers performed at the same level as normally developing second graders, which was nowhere near mastery.

Thirdly, by expanding the morpheme analysis task, it was found that language-disabled second graders and adult poor readers were more successful in analyzing two-syllable than one-syllable word pairs. For these subjects, two-syllable words may have proven easier than one-syllable words because the syllabic boundaries coincided with the morphemic segments, suggesting that the experimental groups are at a serious disadvantage when faced with the task of analyzing the morphemic structure of monosyllabic words.

Finally, it is notable that, even though most of the subjects demonstrated their implicit knowledge of the past tense rule on the *Berry—Talbott*, only those subjects with high overall performance on this task showed some degree of proficiency when explicitly analyzing the internal morphemic structure of past tense words. In contrast, the subjects who performed poorly on the *Berry—Talbott* were relatively unable to analyze the internal morphemic structure of the past tense words, and omitted relatively more past tense inflectional morphemes in writing. Yet they too were able to use the morphological rule for past tense on the *Berry—Talbott*. This pattern of performance suggests that it is the lack of explicit awareness of morphemic structure that should cause us the most concern. Although these subjects demonstrated some ability to manipulate phonemic structure, based on the errors made on the morpheme analysis task, they did not seem to understand further that inflected words are composed of groups of phonemes that form morphemes. Therefore, it seems probable that their lack of explicit understanding of morphophonemic structure, in conjunction with their generally weak implicit knowledge of the morphology, account in large measure for the morphemic errors they make in writing.

It seems clear, then, that even at the primary level, if children are to develop good written language skills, it is not enough for them to understand that words are made up of phonemic segments. Previous research into the spelling and written expression performance of older children and adults with learning problems demonstrated that errors on inflected and derived forms of words are a major characteristic of their written products. The research presented here provides further evidence of morphemic errors in writing and suggests that such errors are highly related to a deficiency at the implicit level, and especially at the explicit level, of morphological knowledge. Therefore, it is of critical importance that we assess the morphological knowledge of young children so that we may identify those who are at risk for learning problems and help them to develop the linguistic skills they need to become proficient at using morphological structures correctly in their written language.

6. EDUCATIONAL IMPLICATIONS

The assessment of morphological knowledge should be part of the evaluation process for children and adults referred because of difficulties with oral or written language production. This assessment, whenever possible, should measure knowledge of the morphology in both elicited production tasks and in samples of spontaneous speech and writing. In spoken language, results obtained on an elicited task such as the *Berry—Talbott* or the *Test for Examining Expressive Morphology* (Shipley *et al.*, 1983) should be compared to results obtained from a spontaneous language sample. Dictated spelling, elicited writing, and spontaneous writing tasks should be administered to determine as fully as possible difficulties in using inflectional morphemes in a variety of writing conditions. Although the use of spontaneous writing samples should yield written output that is the most similar to the student's written products outside of the evaluation setting, this type of task will only be useful if a sufficient amount of output is generated for analysis. Finally, since this study demonstrates that explicit analysis of the morphemic structure of spoken works may be deficient even when expressive use of those structures is intact, tasks that measure awareness of a wide range of morphological structures in both mono-syllabic and multisyllabic word pairs should be developed and used.

In order to best help our students, it seems a necessary first step to teach them to use grammatical morphemes correctly in their spoken language, if they are not doing so already. To accomplish this most effectively, target morphemes should be modelled, emphasized, and elicited as often as possible in naturalistic, rather than strictly clinical, settings. To consolidate correct use of these structures, it is essential to teach students to monitor their own productions so that they will learn to correct their errors and eventually master each target. Techniques that facilitate self-monitoring require that the students, begin to develop some explicit awareness of the morphemic structure of words. These techniques include (1) providing the rule that is needed to inflect the word correctly, (2) giving the choice of correct and incorrect versions of the word, (3) repeating back the person's error with a questioning intonation, and (4) pointedly withholding any form of response when an error has been made.

In the majority of cases, however, the major focus of morphological training should be at a more explicit level. The present results suggest that it is critical to teach these children and adults to become explicitly aware of the morphemic structure of spoken words. It is this explicit awareness of their language that should help them to apprehend the internal structure of the new words that they are required to read and spell. Furthermore, our results with adult poor readers demonstrate that *direct* teaching of this skill is essential, since extensive exposure to language, traditional forms of instruction, and maturation are not sufficient to ensure the development of adequate morphological knowledge.

To facilitate the development of morpheme analysis skills, our results suggest that two-syllable inflected words should be introduced before one-syllable words. For example, it may be easier to teach students to isolate the base word *help* from the inflected form *helping* than from the inflected forms *helped* and *helps*, since the morphemic boundaries of the word *helping* correspond to its syllabic boundaries. Of course, it will be important not to restrict this teaching entirely to bisyllabic words, or students may succeed only because they acquire the ability to segment words into their syllabic units without truly developing any sensitivity to the corresponding morphemic units. Therefore, monosyllabic inflected words should be introduced as soon as possible. They could be incorporated easily into the structural analysis process described by Elkonin (1977). That is, in addition to teaching students to analyze the spoken word *hat* into its phonemic segments by using plastic counters to represent each segment, we could also teach them to analyze the inflected form *hats*.

While doing so, we can explain the function of the plural morpheme and, by contrasting the singular and plural forms in pictures, with counters, and finally with letters, we can illustrate the importance of accurately representing both base and inflectional morphemes in written language.

When teaching spelling and reading, beginning instruction should focus on the development of structural analysis skills at both the morphemic and phonemic levels. It is clear that children should be taught that words (whether they are spoken, read, or spelled) are composed of morphemes, which, in turn, are composed of phonemes. Instruction should proceed from the analysis of spoken words, as discussed above, using procedures similar to those outlined by Elkonin (1977) and Blachman (1984), to the addition of alphabetic letters to represent the phonemic (and morphemic) segments of each word. After each word is written, students should be instructed to read it aloud and to check the spelling. Once a small corpus of words is acquired, in both base and inflected forms, it will be necessary to teach some common irregular words such as *the, a, some, is, are, I*, and *have*, so that sentence writing can be introduced. Next, students should be instructed to formulate grammatically correct phrases and sentences using the words they have been taught (and others with similar orthographic patterns). For example, sentences could include "I have a hat", "I have hats", "The cat is black", and "The cats are black". After the sentence has been produced orally, students can attempt to write it, read it back, and check for spelling. Throughout this process, the emphasis should be on completely representing both the base words and their inflectional morphemes, and on self-monitoring one's productions to ensure that errors are detected and corrections are made, or at least attempted. Although aspects of this process will need modification for older children and adults, the goal of increasing sensitivity to the morphemic structure of words should not be altered.

In addition to this type of training, less structured writing and reading activities, such as creative story or journal writing and oral reading of connected text, should be incorporated into the instructional program. These will aid the teacher in measuring the generalization of those skills taught in structural analysis lessons to more spontaneous tasks.

In conclusion, the research presented in this chapter constitutes the initial stage in an ongoing examination of the relationship of levels of morphological knowledge in spoken language to the ability to represent morphemes in writing. In the future, we need to study in greater depth those children, adolescents, and adults who demonstrate written language difficulties. In this way, we can continue to document deficiencies in sensitivity to morphophonemic structure, and further improve our diagnostic and instructional procedures for these groups.

REFERENCES

Anderson, P. L.: 1982, 'A preliminary study of syntax in the written expression of learning disabled children', *Journal of Learning Disabilities* **15**, 359—362.
Berko, J.: 1958, 'The child's learning of English morphology', *Word* **14**, 150—177.
Berry, M. and Talbott: 1966, *Berry—Talbott Language Test: Comprehension of Grammar*, Rockford, Ill.
Blachman, B.: 1983, 'Are we assessing the linguistic factors critical in early reading?', *Annals of Dyslexia* **33**, 91—109.
Blachman, B.: 1984, 'Language analysis skills and early reading acquisition', in G. Wallach and K. Butler (eds.), *Language-Learning Disabilities in School-Age Children*, Williams and Wilkins, Baltimore.
Brittain, M.: 1970, 'Inflectional performance and early reading achievement', *Reading Research Quarterly* **6**, 34—48.
Brown, R.: 1973, *A First Language: The Early Stages*, Harvard University Press, Cambridge, Mass.
Chomsky, N. and Halle, M.: 1968, *The Sound Pattern of English*, Harper and Row, New York.
Cicci, R.: 1980, 'Written language disorders', *Bulletin of The Orton Society* **30**, 240—251.
Derwing, B. and Baker, W.: 1977, 'The psychological basis for morphological rules', in J. McNamara (ed.), *Language Learning and Thought*, Academic Press, New York.
Derwing, B. and Baker, W.: 1979, 'Recent research on the acquisition of English morphology', in P. Fletcher and M. Garman (eds.), *Language Acquisition*, Cambridge University Press, Cambridge.
deVilliers, J. and deVilliers, P.: 1973, 'A cross-sectional study of the acquisition of grammatical morphemes', *Journal of Psycholinguistic Research* **2**, 267—278.
Doehring, D., Trites, R., Patel, P. and Fiedorowicz, C.: 1981, *Reading Disabilities: The Interaction of Reading, Language, and Neuropsychological Deficits*, Academic Press, New York.
Dunn, L. M. and Smith, J. O.: 1965, *Peabody Language Development Kits*, American Guidance Service, Circle Pines, Minn.
Elkonin, D. B.: 1977, 'USSR', in J. Downing (ed.), *Comparative Reading*, Macmillan, New York.
Fischer, F. W.: 1980, 'Spelling proficiency and sensitivity to linguistic structure', unpublished doctoral dissertation, University of Connecticut.
Fox, B. and Routh, D.: 1980, 'Phoneme analysis and severe reading disability in children', *Journal of Psycholinguistic Research* **9**, 115—119.
Gregg, N.: 1983, 'College learning disabled writer: Error patterns and instructional alternatives', *Journal of Learning Disabilities* **16** (6), 334—338.
Hanson, V. L., Shankweiler, D. and Fischer, F. W.: 1983, 'Determinants of spelling ability in deaf and hearing adults: Access to linguistic structure', *Cognition* **14**, 323—344.
Liberman, I. Y.: 1971, 'Basic research in speech and lateralization of language: Some implications for reading disability', *Bulletin of the Orton Society* **21**, 71—87.
Liberman, I. Y.: 1973, 'Segmentation of the spoken word and reading acquisition', *Bulletin of the Orton Society* **23**, 65—77.
Liberman, I. Y.: 1983, 'A language-oriented view of reading and its disabilities', in H. R. Myklebust (ed.), *Progress in Learning Disabilities*, Vol. V, Grune and Stratton, New York.
Liberman, I. Y., Liberman, A. M., Mattingly, I. G. and Shankweiler, D.: 1980, 'Orthography and the beginning reader', in J. Kavanaugh and R. Venezky (eds.), *Orthography, Reading, & Dyslexia*, University Park Press, Baltimore, MD.
Liberman, I. Y., Rubin, H., Duques, S. and Carlisle, J.: 1985, 'Linguistic abilities and

spelling proficiency in kindergarteners and adult poor spellers', in D. B. Gray and J. F. Kavanaugh, *Biobehavioral Measures of Dyslexia*, York Press, Parkton, MD.

Liberman, I. Y., Shankweiler, D., Fischer, F. W. and Carter, B.: 1974, 'Explicit syllable and phoneme segmentation in the young child', *Journal of Experimental Child Psychology* **18**, 201—212.

Lundberg, I., Olofsson, A. and Wall, S.: 1980, 'Reading and spelling skills in the first school years predicted from phoneme awareness skills in kindergarten', *Scandinavian Journal of Psychology* **21**, 159—173.

Mattingly, I. G.: 1972, 'Reading, the linguistic process, and linguistic awareness', in J. F. Kavanaugh and I. G. Mattingly, *Language by Ear and by Eye*, The MIT Press, Cambridge, MA.

Moran, M. R.: 1981, A comparison of formal features of written language of learning disabled, low-achieving and achieving secondary students (Research Report No. 34), University of Kansas Institute for Research in Learning Disabilities, Lawrence, Kansas.

Myklebust, H.: 1973, *Development and Disorders of Written Language: Studies of Normal and Exceptional Children*, Vol. 2, Grune and Stratton, New York.

Perin, D.: 1983, 'Phonemic segmentation and spelling', *British Journal of Psychology* **74**, 129—144.

Read, C.: 1971, 'Pre-school children's knowledge of English phonology', *Harvard Educational Review* **41**, 1—34.

Read, C.: 1975, 'Children's categorizations of speech sounds in English', NCTE Committee on Research Report No. 17 (Urbana, Illinois), Eric Document Reproduction Service No. Ed 112, 426.

Rubin, H.: 1984, 'An investigation of the development of morphological knowledge and its relationship to early spelling ability', unpublished doctoral dissertation, University of Connecticut.

Rubin, H.: 1985, [Follow-up study of morphological knowledge in relation to performance on spontaneous and dictated written expression tasks.] Unpublished raw data.

Rubin, H.: 1987, 'The development of morphological knowledge in relation to early spelling ability', Haskins Laboratories Status Report on Speech Research, SR-89/90, 121—131.

Rubin, H., Patterson, P., & Kantor, M. (in press). Morphological development and writing ability in children and adults. *Language, Speech, and Hearing Services in Schools*.

Selby, S.: 1972, 'The development of morphological rules in children', *British Journal of Educational Psychology* **42**, 293—299.

Shipley, K. G., Stone, T. A. and Sue, M. B.: 1983, *Test for Examining Expressive Morphology*, Communication Skill Builders, Tucson, Arizona.

Szolusha, C., Messineo, L. V., Lucas, E., Roseff, S., Lasher, B., Carriera, K., Wyland, J. and Humphrey, W.: 1984, *Spelling Steps and Strategies*. Unpublished program. (Available from C. Szolusha, Parker Memorial School, 104 Old Post Road, Tolland, CT.)

Templin, M.: 1957, *Certain Language Skills in Children: Their Development and Interrelationships*, University of Minnesota Press, Minneapolis.

Treiman, R. and Baron, J.: 1981, 'Segmental analysis ability: Development and relation to reading ability', in G. E. MacKinnon and T. G. Waller (eds.), *Reading Research: Advances in Theory and Practice*, Vol. 3, Academic Press, New York.

Vogel, S.: 1975, *Syntactic Abilities in Normal and Dyslexic Children*, University Park Press, Baltimore.

Vogel, S.: 1983, 'A qualitative analysis of morphological development in learning disabled and achieving children', *Journal of Learning Disabilities* **16**, 416—420.

Wiig, E., Semel, E. and Crouse, M.: 1973, 'The use of morphology by high-risk and learning disabled children', *Journal of Learning Disabilities* **6**, 457—465.

Zifcak, M.: 1981, 'Phonological awareness and reading acquisition', *Contemporary Educational Psychology* **6**, 117—126.

APPENDIX 1

Examples of Elicited Writing Responses

High second grade

1. The girl raked a pile of leaves.

2. The boy cleaned the shelfs

3. The girl ironed the dress.

4. The girl made a cake.

5. The boy fixed the toys.

6. The girl kicked the ball.

7. The hourses jumped over the fence.

8. The girl climded the tree.

9. The girls picked some flowers.

10. The girl washed the cloese.

Low second grade

1. She racket all the leves.

2. He wash the dichas.

3. She icnd It.

4. She dak a cake.

5. he madit,

6. She kick it,

7. They jum it,

8. She cill m it,

9. They pik it,

10. She wash them

High first grade

1. The gril raked the tears.

2. The picked up the cups and plates

3. The gril lyred the shert s

4. The gril cookedthe cake.

5. The boy fixed the toys.

6. The gril kiced the ball,

7. The housees jumed over the fens.

8. The gril climded the tree.

9. The grils picked the flouws

10. The gril wost the clothes.

Low first grade

The girl rack the levs.

The box drid the dich

She I ngro

She cukt the cake

He mad to cars.

The girl chek the ball.

Hors jumt

The girl clim up the tree.

The girls peck the flors.

the girl wrst the clos.

APPENDIX 2

Spontaneous Writing Samples

High second grade

The creature

One night a little boy named Bobby was sleeping. All of a sudden he woke up somone or somthing was at his house that didn't belong there! Then he saw something else! Foot prints on the wall! Now ofcorse it wasin't a person people don't have claws! This thing did. if he made footprints that must of ment he steped in the mud outside his window. He ran to his mom & Dad's room and said

"Mommy, Daddy thears a monster in my room!" Mommy said, "Realy hunny go back to bed! Mom wont you just come see? Ohh all right. When they got in the room mommy almost fainted! But gladely she did not! Honey I'm sory what I said but I thought there was no such thing! Bobby said, "Ohh, thats ok now all we have to do is find him!" I'll go get daddy he was under the covers he had seen the monster he was under the bed!

Mommy said," Don't be a big old sissy. Go get him he's under the bed! Ohh all right. He caught he monster. The next day they brought him to the pound he never came back again

Low second grade

A dare brok ther the Winlo
And Klim up the
Wall and ate the
Cun in
And the dog star
et to bark And

woek   up the doy And

The doy statered

to   srem   and evy

for   his   mom and dad

And   his   dad   called

the   plessr

the end

High first grade

I think that   a   rackoon
broke the window   and left
some foot prints and the dog
is nirvis and the boy is
scard that a bear snuk in
and that his mother is going
to be veary mad and if the
boy finds the anmal that
broke the window I bet
the dog is going to kill the
anmal because dogs don't
like others anmals and if
the dog is a baby german
sheperd it will be a good fight
and I bet the baby german

sheperd will win because
german sheperds have sharp
teeth and a rackoon is
tuph too but I still think
the german sheperd.

Low first grade.

A monst came in my rom I saw some
foot print on my wol I saw in the
nite my window was cracdd I had a dog
he sow it to we went out to fined it
we didt find it thene we foned it
then we lost it then we fond it was
are pet dwe had funs with it
I played with it and my dog
did to.

APPENDIX 3

Spontaneous Writing Sample of an Adult Poor Reader

The boy and his dog were a sleep.

When a bar crashed thou the windol

The boy and his dog jup.

The dog bark and the bar ran

up the ~~t~~ wall. The boy cried and
the dog barked more and more.
.Untill the bar ran out the windol.
The boy's mother and father came running,
to his room. ~~E~~ The boys mother
~~grew~~ helded ~~the~~ him and father
chack the house,

ALFONSO CARAMAZZA AND ARGYE E. HILLIS

MODULARITY: A PERSPECTIVE FROM THE ANALYSIS OF ACQUIRED DYSLEXIA AND DYSGRAPHIA[1]

1. WEAK MODULARITY

A central canon of the cognitive and the neural sciences is that even the simplest behavior reflects the concerted activity of a complex set of processes — processes that may be given independent characterizations. On this view, cognitive and neural systems are assumed to be *modular*, in the information processing sense used in cognitive psychology (Simon, 1962) and cognitive neuroscience (Marr, 1976). We can schematically represent this general hypothesis as follows: I $\rightarrow$ $\{P_1, P_2, \ldots, P_i, \ldots, P_n\}$ $\rightarrow$ O, where I and O are input and output, respectively, and P stands for cognitive or neural process. Depending on the level of theoretical development in particular domains of neuroscience or cognitive science, the p's in some I/O function will be more or less structured and detailed. For example, there is now considerable appreciation of the general principles that govern the neurophysiological processes that characterize sensory and motor activity (see Mountcastle, 1978, for discussion), but little understanding of the neurophysiological mechanisms involved in language processing. Analogously, at the computational level there is increasingly deeper understanding of the component processes that comprise linguistic ability (see Chomsky, 1986, for discussion), but little understanding of the mechanisms that subserve mathematical reasoning.

Consider briefly the familiar case of the visual system. A number of properties of this system are well known. It now seems clear (primarily through the work of Hubel and Wiesel, but also Zeki and others) that the visual cortex has a richly structured organization. Sets of simple cells (i.e., cells that respond to relatively "simple" stimulus patterns) connect to complex cells, and in turn, sets of complex cells connect to hypercomplex cells. Architecturally, these cell types are not only segregated by gross neuroanatomical area but also have local neuroanatomical structure. Thus, simple cells are organized into functionally homogeneous columns; within these columns there are complex cells that receive direct connections from the simple cells; and, in turn, columns are organized into hypercolumns consisting of sets of columns which analyze lines of all orientations from a particular region in space for both eyes. In short, the projections from the lateral geniculate body through the peristriate cortex are assumed to represent a functionally hierarchical system: low-level analyzers converge on progressively higher, more abstract analyzers.

Here we wish to emphasize two aspects of this general conception of

R. M. Joshi (ed.), Written Language Disorders, 71—84.
© 1991 *Kluwer Academic Publishers. Printed in the Netherlands.*

the organization of the visual system: (1) a complex function such as vision may be analyzed into a set of distinct neurophysiological subprocesses — the P's in our schematic equation for relating input to output; and (2) selective damage to the neurophysiological subprocesses that comprise the visual system should result in distinctive functional disorders of visual processing. A more general characterization of this latter point is useful to us here: to the extent to which the neural mechanisms that subserve a complex function consist of neuroanatomically and/or neurophysiologically distinguishable processing units, it is possible to selectively damage these processing units resulting in functionally distinctive patterns of perceptual or cognitive impairment.

Consider now an analogous example from cognitive psychology — the lexical system. Figure 1 shows a highly schematic representation of the lexical processes involved in reading and writing. There is considerable support for the view that lexical information is represented in distinct modality-specific lexical components, separately for input and output processes. Recent research on the lexical system has assumed a componential structure and has focused on aspects of the internal structure of the hypothesized components — for example, on the issue of whether the output of the Orthographic Output Lexicon consists of morphemic or whole-word representations. Thus, as in the case of the visual system, one of the leading hypotheses in research on the lexical system is that the complex activity of word processing in such tasks as reading and writing may be analyzed into a set of distinct processes — once again the P's in our schematic equation for relating input to output.

In the context of a componential analysis of cognitive or neural functions, a crucial issue concerns the nature of the criteria and arguments used to motivate a particular parse of a complex function into a set of independent processes. Although there are some important differences between the criteria used by neurophysiologists and cognitive psychologists in motivating their respective componential analyses, the similarities are much more striking and significant. In both cases the postulation of a distinction between two processes is based on the assumption that there are general principles that apply at one level of analysis but not at another, or that the form of representation involved at one level of analysis is different from that involved at another level of analysis. For example, the cognitive mechanism referred to as "Orthographic Output Lexicon" is distinguished from other mechanisms principally on the basis of the type of representation it takes as input (semantic) and the type of representation it computes for output (graphemic). Obviously, there are other (empirical) features which may serve to distinguish between hypothesized components of processing. One such feature is whether a component of processing is subject to selective disruption under conditions of brain damage. In this paper we focus on evidence of this latter type to address

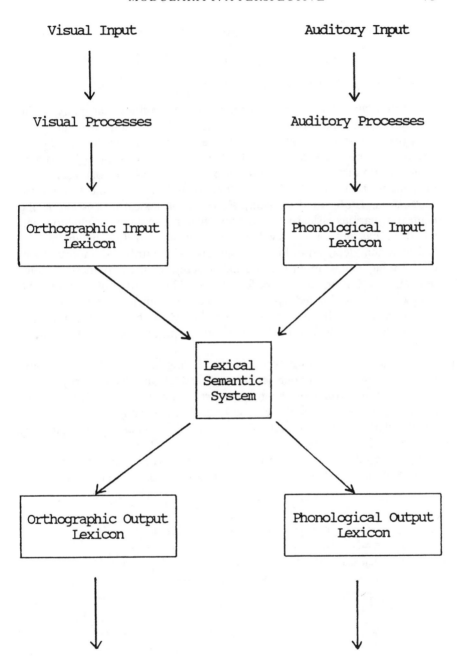

Fig. 1. Schematic representation of the lexical system.

issues about cognitive architecture, specifically in the context of the lexical system.

2. PROCESSING COMPONENTS AS MODULES

We shall assume familiarity with the basic assumptions that motivate the use of impaired performance resulting from brain damage to infer the structure of normal cognitive systems, and simply assert that damage to any one of the mechanisms involved in lexical processing will result in some discriminable form of lexical processing dysfunction, each form presumably reflecting the locus of functional damage to the system (see Caramazza, 1986, for discussion). Research on lexical processing, in the context of various tasks such as reading, naming, sentence production, and so forth, has not only provided empirical support for the distributed lexical system depicted in Figure 1 but has also contributed importantly in constraining claims about the internal structure of the hypothesized components (see Caramazza, 1988, for review). This rich literature cannot be reviewed in the limited space available here. Instead, for illustrative purposes, we briefly discuss some of the research carried out in our laboratory which speaks to the question of the modular organization of the lexicon.

Consider a well-known type of oral reading error produced by some patients — semantic paralexic error (Marshall and Newcombe, 1973). Table 1 shows some of the reading errors produced by K.E., a well-educated, 52-year-old male who suffered left-hemisphere brain damage. (A detailed description and analysis of this patient's performance is reported in Hillis, Rapp, Romani & Caramazza, 1990.)

What could be the basis for these strange errors and what must we assume about the structure of the reading process, and more specifically

TABLE 1
Examples of K.E.'s semantic paralexic errors

Stimulus	Response
apple	orange
shirt	socks
screw	hammer
nail	pliers
fork	knife
wrist	ear
bed	couch
leopard	lion
rocket	airplane

the structure of the lexical system, in order to explain the occurrence of these errors? Various efforts to explain the occurrence of these errors have located the source of the problem at the level of access to the semantic system, or at the level of the semantic system itself, or at the level of the Ouput Phonological Lexicon (see Coltheart, Patterson & Marshall, 1980, for discussion). (More "complex" explanations have appealed to the intervention of "right-hemisphere mechanisms" called into service as a result of damage to the left hemisphere. We shall ignore this type of explanation in this discussion.)

TABLE 2

Examples of K.E.'s semantic errors in oral naming

Stimulus	Response
nail	screw
hammer	pliers
wrist	foot
leopard	tiger
sock	gloves
dolphin	whale

Suppose, however, that we were to test K.E. in a picture-naming task and we found that he also made semantic errors in this task — errors such as these shown in Table 2. Indeed, upon testing K.E. in a tactile naming task (i.e., naming objects by touch only) and upon analysis of his spontaneous speech production, we discover that he makes semantic errors in all tasks involving speech production, irrespective of the modality of stimulus input (see Tables 3 and 4). These results allow us to reject the hypothesis that the semantic paralexic errors produced by K.E. reflect damage to modality-specific *input* mechanisms, and would initially appear to suggest that the locus of deficit is at the level of the Phonological

TABLE 3

Examples of K.E.'s semantic errors in a tactile naming task

Stimulus	Response
glove	sock
nail	hammer
tie	belt
sponge	towel
fork	knife
spatula	sponge

TABLE 4

Examples of K.E.'s semantic errors in his spontaneous speech

Speech produced	Intended production
driving . . . tomorrow	I drove yesterday
sore throat	sore tooth
good night	good morning
phone . . . Pam (daughter)	call Amy (wife)
eat . . . coffee	drink coffee

Output Lexicon. However, other analyses of K.E.'s performance allow us to further restrict the possible locus of damage to the semantic system itself.

K.E.'s performance in writing tasks — writing to dictation and written naming, to both visually and tactually presented objects — was also characterized by the presence of semantic errors (see Table 5).

The occurrence of semantic paragraphias in these tasks undermines the hypothesis that the semantic errors produced by K.E. result from selective damage to an *output* lexicon. Further evidence against an explanation in terms of an output deficit was obtained from auditory and visual word comprehension tasks, where K.E. showed difficulties in lexical semantic processing comparable to those shown in production tasks. For example, when the same 144 items that gave rise to frequent semantic errors (about 30% of total responses) on reading, writing, and naming tasks were presented in word-picture matching tasks, about 30% of K.E.'s responses were semantic errors. The converging results of all of these tasks strongly

TABLE 5

Examples of K.E.'s semantic errors in various writing tasks

Stimulus	Writing to dictation	Written naming (pictures)	Written naming (tactile)
fork			knife
sock	mittens		
stapler	scissors	paper	paper clip
mitten	pocket		
elbow	tooth		
spatula	pan	sponge	sponge
nose	finger		
screw		nail	
tape	pencil	clip	paper
glove		mitten	mitten
wrist		leg	

argue for the hypothesis that the locus of functional lesion responsible for the observed pattern of dysfunction in K.E. is at the level of the semantic system itself.

The analysis of K.E.'s performance provides compelling evidence in favor of the hypothesis that the input and output, modality-specific lexicons — where phonological and orthographic information are represented and where, presumably, morphological and syntactic information are also represented — are interconnected through a single, modality-independent lexicon. The alternative, modality-specific semantics hypothesis, forcefully defended most recently by Shallice (1987), is undermined by K.E.'s pattern of performance. There are some results, however, which have been interpreted as favoring the modality-specific semantics hypothesis. One such type of result is the dissociation of semantic errors by modality of input or output.

Consider the performance of two patients (R.G.B. and H.W.) we have recently had the opportunity to evaluate on a number of lexical-processing tasks (a detailed analysis of the performance by these patients is reported in Caramazza and Hillis, 1990). Like K.E., these patients made frequent semantic paralexias following left hemisphere strokes. However, the pattern of performance by these patients across tasks involving a variety of input and output modalities (Table 6) turns out to be quite different from that of K.E. As is readily apparent from the table, the two patients are unimpaired in comprehension tasks but are moderately impaired in tasks that require spoken production (despite quite fluent spontaneous speech). Although both patients had severe spelling difficulties, the crucial aspect in these data for present purposes is the fact that they produce semantic errors in only one output modality — spoken production. A better

TABLE 6
Performance across tasks on the same 47 items (given in percent of total responses)

Task	R.G.B.		H.W.	
	Semantic errors	Omissions or unrecognizable responses	Semantic errors	Omissions or unrecognizable responses
Oral naming: pictures	36%	2%	34%	4%
Oral naming: tactile	36%	0%	36%	9%
Oral reading	32%	2%	34%	4%
Written naming	0%	6%	0%	2%
Dictation	0%	6%	0%	4%
Auditory word — picture matching	0%	0%	0%	0%
Printed word — picture matching	0%	0%	0%	0%

appreciation of these patients' performance is achieved if we consider qualitative aspects of their performance.

Tables 7 and 8 show examples of the two patients' performance on the oral reading, oral-naming and written-naming tasks. A striking feature of these patients' performance is that even when they fail to access the correct lexical-phonological form, it is apparent (despite spelling errors)

TABLE 7
Examples of R.G.B.'s responses in oral vs. written production tasks

Stimulus	Oral reading	Oral naming	Written naming
sock	stocking	mitten	sock
pear	apple	fruit ... banana	pear
cap	hat	stocking	cap
dish	plate	jar ... cup	jar
pan	cook on a stove	stove ... dish	pan
pot	pan	cup ... saucer	pot
plug	put in something ... to stop it up	outlet	plug
kangaroo	giraffe	racoon	kag oo
dolphin	water pelican	florida ... fish	d l p
donkey	monkey	monkey	dokey
lemon	lime	sour	lemon
celery	lettuce	lettuce	celey
squash	pumpkin, no	melon, no, what you eat ...	sq s
goose	thing that flies	turkey	goose
camel	hump	water stored up in his back	caml

TABLE 8
Examples of H.W.'s errors in oral vs. written production tasks

Stimulus	Oral reading	Oral naming	Written naming
lime	lemon	melon	lime
fork	eat	spoon	fork
tie	neck	belt	tie
jar	lunch	bottle	jar
razor	shave	shaver	razor
octopus	clam	squid	octop
leopard	cat	cat	l ap d
shelf	top	book	shef
cheek	cheek	feet	chek
ankles	arm	feet	a kns
mustache	scalp	beard	mutac
finger	ring	ring	figre
thumb	tongue	wrist	thub

that they nonetheless can access the correct lexical-orthographic form. Thus, for example, they might say jacket for shirt but will attempt to write shirt.

Other evidence allows us to establish unequivocally that the patients *know* the meaning of the word they are unable to produce orally and produce instead a semantically related word. When R.G.B. and H.W. are asked to define the words they make semantic errors to, immediately following the errors, they define them correctly. Examples of the two patients' performance in this task are shown in Table 9. Finally, it is important to note that on repeated testing of reading or naming, the patients as often as not produced the correct response to items that previously elicited semantic errors. They also frequently produced semantic errors to previously correct items. In other words, the correct response is available to the patient, but it is sometimes inaccessible.

The pattern of results described for R.G.B. and H.W. allows the conclusion that in each case the lexical-semantic system is intact and that the source of their semantic errors must be located at the level of the Phonological Output Lexicon. The fact that both reading and auditory comprehension were unimpaired also allows the conclusion that the Phonologic and Orthographic Input Lexicons are intact, even for words that could not be retrieved for verbal output. That is, even though an

TABLE 9
R.G.B.'s and H.W.'s definitions of words following semantic errors

Oral Reading

Stimulus	Response	Definition
R.G.B.		
records	radio	you play 'em on a phonograph . . .
		can also mean notes you take and keep
tomato	salad	you get 'em in the summer
		Jackie used to grow 'em . . .
		same color as apples
necklace	necktie	you would wear
		a woman would have around her neck . . .
		made out of metal . . . gold or silver
airport	airplane	where they're . . . airplanes are parked . . .
		where you go to get on the plane at
H.W.		
scramble	fry	instead of in order, it's all mixed up
interest	bank	you go to the bank and put it in and
		you get more money . . . not very much now
village	live	small city
history	school	find out things how they used to be

orally presented word consistently accessed the corresponding phonological representation, which in turn addressed semantic information, the same phonological representation could not be consistently accessed for output. This result provides strong support for the hypothesis that phonological information is represented or accessed separately for input and output processes.

(Parenthetically, the opposite type of dissociation to the one just described — the production of semantic errors restricted to the written output modality — has also been recorded. Although we do not have as detailed a set of observations as those reported for R.G.B. and H.W., we have observed a patient (N.H.) who makes semantic paragraphic errors but no semantic errors in lexical-processing tasks involving spoken output. Some examples of her semantic paragraphias are shown in Table 10.)

TABLE 10
Examples of N.H.'s semantic errors in written production tasks

Stimulus	Dictation	Naming
bring	carry	
house plant		flowers
thumb		finger
open	close	

The contrasting results between K.E. on the one hand, and R.G.B. and H.W. on the other, strongly constrain the kinds of claims we can make about the functional architecture of the lexical system. It would appear that we must assume: (1) that there is a modality-independent semantic system — the system selectively damaged in patient K.E.; and (2) that there are modality-specific output lexicons in which lexical-phonological and lexical-orthographic information are represented — the two systems shown to be dissociable in patients R.G.B. and H.W. Additionally, we must assume that there are functionally independent input and output lexicons in which lexical-phonological information is represented, since this information was consistently accessed for input, but inconsistently for output, by R.G.B. and H.W.

It should not go unnoted that the experimental evidence adduced to constrain claims about the functional architecture of the lexical system comes to us through the analysis of performance of complex tasks such as reading, sentence comprehension, and so forth. Indeed, the interpretation of some pattern of impaired performance as relevant to claims about the lexical system presupposes a model of the task used to obtain the performance from which inferences about the lexical system are drawn. Thus, for example, if a patient were to make some type of spelling error that we wished to interpret as evidence for morphological decomposition in the Orthographic Output Lexicon we would have to rule out the possibility that that type of error could reflect the functioning of some other component of processing in the spelling system. This situation naturally explains why in cognitive neuropsychology so much emphasis is placed on the need to develop models of the complex tasks used to obtain patients' performance. Necessity has been turned into a virtue: there is a healthy emphasis on the development of models of cognitively complex tasks. These models are also "modular" in the sense that they consist of sets of independent processing components.

Consider as an example the spelling system, or more precisely, that part of the spelling system that concerns the computation of a graphemic representation for motor output. There is now considerable evidence that the functional architecture of the spelling system is roughly as shown in Figure 2. That is, we have strong evidence for a "modular" spelling system consisting of a set of processing mechanisms in addition to the lexical components discussed earlier.

Grant us for the moment that the results we have described (but there are others which strongly converge with those presented here) support the hypothesis of a distributed lexical system consisting of a modality-independent lexical semantic component and modality-specific input and output components. What are the implications of this conclusion, if any, for Fodor's (1983) recent characterization of mind as a modular system? More precisely, are the hypothesized modality-specific lexical components reasonable candidates for the status of "module" in Fodor's sense of this term? What about the other components of processing involved in spelling (or reading, sentence production, and so forth)? Can these components of processing be ascribed the status of "module"?

3. ON FODORIAN MODULARITY

Fodor has proposed a set of criteria for distinguishing between modular and nonmodular systems. Processing systems that have the properties of domain specificity, processing mandatoriness, information encapsulation, speed, lack of access by other systems to intermediate representations, shallow output, neural localization, susceptibility to characteristic breakdown, and characteristic pace and sequencing of ontogeny are considered to be modular. Although Fodor has taken the position that modularity may be a matter of degree — the degree of modularity being determined by the number of criteria for modularity that are met by a processing unit — he considers the criterion of information encapsulation (or impenetrability in Pylyshyn's (1984) formulation) to be the most important, and perhaps even defining, in deciding whether a processing "unit" is to be considered a module.

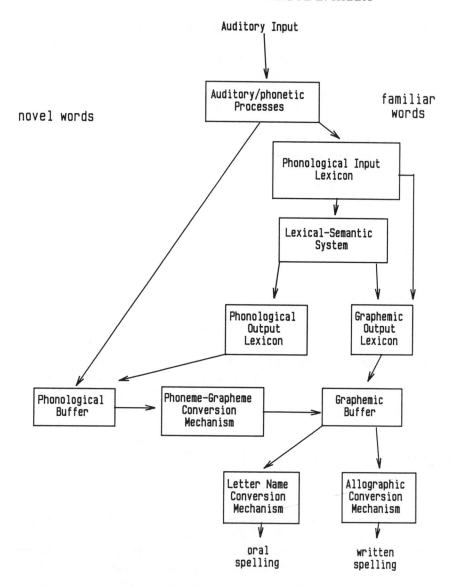

Fig. 2. Schematic diagram of the spelling process.

On Fodor's analysis of various processing systems, the most likely candidates for modularity are the input systems — systems that mediate between "low level" sensory representations (the output of transducers, in Fodor's terms) and central processes involved in belief fixation. Candidate examples of input sytems include mechanisms for color perception, mechanisms for face recognition, mechanisms that assign grammatical descriptions to utterances, and so forth. Finally, although Fodor focuses on input systems in his discussion of likely candidates for modularity he leaves open the possibility that output systems might also be modular.

It should be clear that Fodor's notion of module is much more restrictive than its common use in cognitive psychology, where this term has been used interchangeably with "component of processing" — a relatively general notion as exemplified by its earlier use in the case of the visual and lexical systems. However, it is not at all clear that the components of processing we have identified in this discussion might not, after all, satisfy Fodor's criteria for modularity.

Consider the case of the output lexicons. Are these domain- and modality-specific components informationally encapsulated (or impenetrable to extraneous information)? From the analysis of patients' performance we have presented it is clear that some patients (such as R.G.B. and H.W.) may be able to exercise their intention to produce a word in one modality while failing to do so in another modality. The failure is not due to a low-level motor incapacity but appears to be related to access limitations of modality-specific representation — lexical-orthographic or lexical-phonological. Our data suggest that the patients' semantic representations are intact, as is their motor output ability. Furthermore, the individual representation in the Orthographic and Phonological Output Lexicons that are inaccessible at one time may be accessible at another time, suggesting an access limitation as opposed to a disruption of the informational content of the orthographic or phonological representations in the two lexicons.

The patients' failure to produce target responses in one modality despite the fact that they *know* what it is they want to produce and the fact that they *can produce* the correct lexical form in another modality reflects a highly localized limitation in the system. The rigidly circumscribed nature of the limitation suggests that the damaged lexical systems is *independent* of other processing mechanisms — as close as we can come in the present context to Fodor's notion of encapsulation. Analogous arguments could be developed for other components of processing in complex functional systems such as, for example, spelling.

To conclude, the neuropsychological literature provides compelling evidence that language, perceptual systems, or other conceptual skills may be selectively affected by brain damage. However, there is also evidence that brain damage may selectively affect sentence production while sparing sentence comprehension, sentence comprehension while sparing sentence production, reading while sparing spelling, spelling while sparing reading, and so forth. Of even greater interest is the fact that the selectivity of functional deficits consequent to brain damage appears to extend to components of processing within complex functional systems — e.g., the Phonological Output Lexicon. Since the selectively damaged components are independent and modality- and domain-specific units of processing, we may want to attribute them the status of "module" in Fodor's sense of this term. If we were to do so, Fodorian modularity would no longer concern only faculties of mind (e.g., musical ability) but the more pedestrian components of processing that presumably underlie complex cognitive functions. Indeed, it could turn out that the only level at which we could meaningfully talk of modularity would be at the level of components of processing and *not* cognitive systems or faculties.

NOTE

[1] The work reported here was supported in part by NIH research grants NS23836 and NS22202 to The Johns Hopkins University, The Seaver Institute and The Lounsbery Foundation. The support of these foundations and agencies is gratefully acknowledged.

REFERENCES

Caramzza, A.: 1986, 'On drawing inferences about the structure of normal cognitive systems from the analysis of patterns of impaired performance: The case for single-patient studies', *Brain and Cognition* **5**, 41—66.

Caramazza, A.: 1988, 'Some aspects of language processing revealed through the analysis of acquired aphasia: The lexical system', *Annual Review of Neuroscience* **11**, 395—421.

Caramazza, A. and Hillis, A.: 1990, 'Where do semantic errors come from?' *Cortex* **26**, 95—122.

Chomsky, N.: 1986, *Language and Problems of Knowledge: The Managua Lectures*, MIT Press, Cambridge, MA.

Coltheart, M., Patterson, K. and Marshall, J. (eds.): 1980, *Deep Dyslexia*, Routledge and Kegan Paul, London.

Fodor, J. A.: 1983, *The Modularity of Mind*, MIT Press, Cambridge, MA.

Hillis, A., Rapp, B., Romani, C. and Caramazza, A.: 1990, 'Selective impairment of semantics in lexical processing', *Cognitive Neuropsychology* **7**, 191—244.

Marr, D.: 1976, 'Early processing of visual information', *Philosophical Transactions of the Royal Society of London* **B 275**, 483—524.

Marshall, J. C. and Newcombe, F.: 1973, 'Patterns of paralexia: A psycholinguistic approach', *Journal of Psycholinguistic Research* **2**, 175—199.

Mountcastle, V. B.: 1978, 'An organizing principle for cerebral functions: The unit module and the distributed system', in G. E. Edelman and V. B. Mountcastle (eds.), *The Mindful Brain: Cortical Organization and the Group-Selective Theory of Higher Brain Function*, MIT Press, Cambridge, MA.

Pylyshyn, Z. W.: 1984, *Computation and Cognition: Toward a Foundation for Cognitive Science*, MIT Press, Cambridge, MA.

Shallice, T.: 1987, 'Impairments of semantic processing: Multiple dissociations', in M. Coltheart, G. Sartori and R. Job (eds.), *The Cognitive Neuropsychology of Language*, LEA, London.

Simon, H. A.: 1962, 'The architecture of complexity', *Proceedings of the American Philosophical Society* **106**, 467—482 (December).

GABRIELE MICELI[1]

ON THE INTERPRETATION OF ACROSS-PATIENT VARIABILITY

Some Mechanisms Underlying Nonlexical Spelling Errors

1. INTRODUCTION

Consider the sets of errors displayed in Table 1. They were produced by three patients who premorbidly were adequate spellers of their language but developed a spelling disorder after sustaining brain damage. At face value, there is a close stimulus—error relationship in all the reported examples. All the incorrect responses are nonwords, and most of them are very close to the stimulus item (they can be construed as letter substitutions, insertions, deletions and transpositions). However, other features of these errors suggest that they might differ under crucial respects. For example, if the incorrect spelling responses are read aloud, the errors produced by I.G.R. "sound very similar" to the stimulus, the errors produced by patient J.G. "sound identical" to the stimulus, and the errors produced by patient L.B. "sound somewhat similar" to the stimulus. Should more relevance be given to the similarities or to the differences observed across patients? A motivated answer to this question can be provided only if the investigation proceeds under explicit assumptions, that unequivocally legitimate the conclusion in favor of one of the two

TABLE 1
Examples of errors produced in written spelling-to-dictation by patients I.G.R., J.G. and L.B.

Patient I.G.R. (Caramazza *et al.,* 1986)

dello (of the, m.sg.) → tello; padre (father) → badre; talora (sometimes) → dallora; ventura (venture) → fentura; ritiene (he thinks) → ridiene; altronde (on the other hand) → altromte; soltanto (only) soltando.

Patient J.G. (Goodman and Caramazza, 1986a)

crisp → krisp; grief → greef; budget → budjet; machine → mashine; leopard → leppard; angry → angery; pity → pitty; threat → thret; marriage → marriage; honest → onest; view → vew; thief → theif; cheer → chere; satire → satier; likely → likley.

Patient L.B. (Caramazza *et al.,* 1987)

socio (associate) → sicio; voluto (wanted) → votuto; verita' (truth) → nerita'; svedese (Swedish) → sredese; valige (bags) → viligie; suolo (ground) → sluolo; solerte (diligent) → solertoe; tempo (time) → tempto; perdi (you lose) → pedi; strada (road) → stada; interno (internal) → inteno; acquisto (purchase) → acquito; lungo (long) → lugno; metodo (method) → medoto; allegro (happy) → allergo; squadra (team) → squarda.

R. M. Joshi (ed.), Written Language Disorders, 85—104.
© 1991 *Kluwer Academic Publishers. Printed in the Netherlands.*

alternatives. The aim of the present chapter is to demonstrate that an explicit cognitive model is a necessary prerequisite for theoretically driven analyses of pathological behavior, and in particular for the principled interpretation of across-subject performance variation.

1.1. *A Theory as a Prerequisite for the Analysis of Across-Subject Variation*

The problem of interpreting the variations of performance observed in cognitively impaired subjects is of critical importance for neuropsychological theories. The investigation of across-patient variations should lead eventually to conclude that observed differences result from distinct patterns of impairment of the cognitive system, or that they are the outcome of a quantitatively (but not qualitatively) different damage to the same functional component(s). It is obvious that either conclusion has important consequences on issues regarding the computational structure of cognitive systems. However, until very few years ago, the theoretical problems posed by the investigation and the interpretation of across-patient performance variation have been neglected in neuropsychological research.

For a long time, the most widely adopted approach to the study of cognitively-impaired subjects has relied on the classification of patients as exemplars of one or other clinical category (e.g., Broca's aphasia, agrammatism, deep dyslexia, etc.), based on the presence of a finite set of pathological observations, that were chosen *a priori* on intuitive criteria. Under a strong version of this approach, all subjects classified as instances of a clinical category are considered to be cognitively homogeneous, that is, affected by damage to the same functional locus (or loci) of the cognitive system. Consequently, across-subject variation is legitimately attributed to random factors, uninteresting with respect to a cognitive theory of the system under exam, and dismissed as irrelevant. Under a weaker version of the traditional approach, it is implicitly acknowledged that clinical categories, defined by a restricted set of arbitrarily chosen observations, allow to group subjects who are only *relatively* homogenous as regards their cognitive impairment.[2] In this case, variation may or may not be considered as relevant, but the decision is clearly unprincipled, since it can be based only on some arbitrary criteria, rather than on theoretical justifications.

In a series of papers, Caramazza and his colleagues (Caramazza, 1986; Caramazza and Badecker 1989; Caramazza and Mc Closkey, 1988) have convincingly argued that this approach is substantially inadequate. A finite set of arbitrarily established observations cannot be used to locate *a priori* lesions in the cognitive system. Quite to the contrary, cognitive lesions can only be located *a posteriori*, based on all the observations that are relevant to confirm hypotheses regarding the presence of damage to one component (or set of components) of the cognitive system and to disconfirm all alternative hypotheses. In this view, what counts as a relevant observation is not based on intuition, but is established by an explicit theory of the cognitive system under exam. In the absence of such a theory, patients who are classified as exemplars of a given clinical category on an *a priori* basis are very likely to be heterogeneous as regards the locus of cognitive impairment (an empirical demonstration of this point has been provided in Miceli *et al.,* 1989).

Consequently, appropriate decisions regarding the theoretical relevance of across-subject variations (as in the case of the errors made by the three patients quoted above) can only begin to be made on the basis of a theoretical background. Contemporary research in cognitive neuropsychology has provided such background for studies of oral and written spelling.

1.2. *A Cognitive Model of Spelling*

In recent years, research on the cognitive neuropsychology of spelling has led to formulate a model that has obtained a large consensus (e.g., Ellis, 1982 and 1989; Margolin, 1984; Miceli, 1989; Patterson, 1989; but see, for a different view, Marcel, 1980; Kay and Marcel, 1981; Henderson, 1982; Campbell, 1983). The model (schematically depicted in Figure 1) includes two functionally independent sets of mechanisms: lexical mechanisms, responsible for accessing orthographic representations in word spelling, and phonological mechanisms, responsible for converting phonemes into graphemes in nonword spelling. When a familiar word has to be spelled, a semantic representation or a phonological representation activates an orthographically coded entry in the Graphemic Output Lexicon. Information is represented in the Graphemic Output Lexicon along a number of dimensions, such as frequency, form class and morphological structure, and is stored in morphologically decomposed form. When a novel word has to be spelled, the corresponding phonological sequence is temporarily stored in a short-term memory system (the Phonological Buffer). Correspondence rules between phonemes and graphemes are sequentially applied to the phonological string stored in the Phonological Buffer, by the Phoneme-to-Grapheme Conversion System. Print-to-sound mappings are represented in this system according to their frequency of occurrence in the language, relative to their occurrence in various syllable positions. Orthographic representations addressed in the Graphemic Output Lexicon and orthographic representations assembled by means of Phoneme-to-Grapheme Conversion Rules are temporarily stored in a short-term memory system (the Graphemic Buffer) for the time needed in order to be converted into sequences of graphs (in written spelling), letter names (in oral spelling) or hand/finger movements (in typing).

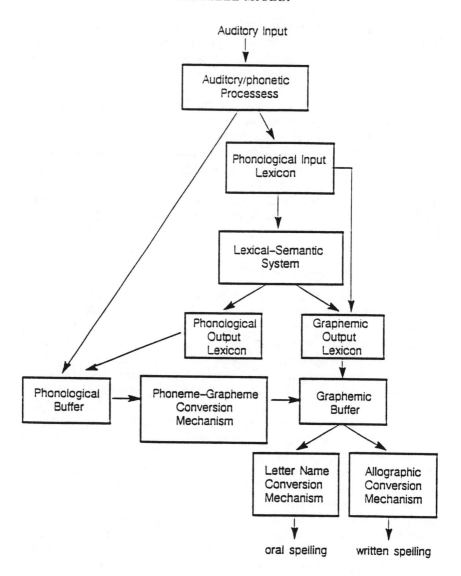

Fig. 1. Schematic diagram of the spelling process.

The model of spelling just presented consists of computational and buffer units, which are included in the functional structure on the basis of theoretical considerations and of empirical evidence. Computational units are required whenever a representation stored in a given code must be converted into a representation stored in a different code. Examples of such units are the Graphemic Output Lexicon, where an orthographic representation is activated by a semantic input, and the Phoneme-to-

Grapheme Conversion System, which maps a sequence of phonemes onto a sequence of graphemes. Buffer systems are included in the functional architecture of a cognitive system when the size of the units that serve as input to a computational component is incommensurate to the size of the units over which that computational component works (Caramazza et al., 1986). The Phonological Buffer and the Grapheme Buffer are examples of such short-term memory components in the spelling system. The Phonological Buffer, used for nonword spelling only, temporarily holds the phonologically coded nonword string prior to its conversion into a graphemic sequence; the Grapheme Buffer, used for both word and nonword spelling, temporarily stores addressed or assembled, orthographically coded strings in preparation for later processing stages. This model, although still underspecified in many respects, offers the theoretical background for fine-grained analyses of spelling disorders.

In performing analyses of acquired cognitive impairments it is assumed that the disorder observed in patients with brain damage transparently results from the normal functioning of the spared components of the model and from the malfunctioning of the disrupted components (Caramazza, 1986). In other words, it is believed that damage to any processing unit of the spelling system results in incorrect responses that transparently reflect the failure of the procedure(s) for which the disrupted unit(s) is responsible in normal subjects. The current knowledge of the procedures that take place in each component of the system provides the theoretical basis necessary to relate a given pattern of pathological performance to the impairment of one or more processing components of the system itself. Thus, both the pattern of spared and impaired performance and the relationships between stimulus and incorrect response can be used to draw inferences on the functional locus of lesion.

Let us now go back to our three subjects. So far, we only know that their errors take the forms exemplified in Table 1. In order to make a principled decision as to whether the errors made by the three patients result from damage to the same processing component or from the impairment of distinct units of the spelling process, a theoretically driven analysis must be performed. To this end, much more needs to be known about the features of the spelling disorder in each patient. In the first place, the full range of the performance obtained by the three patients in spelling and spelling-related tasks must be considered. Secondly, the relationships between stimulus items and incorrect spelling responses must be carefully analyzed.

2. COMPARISON OF THE PATTERNS OF SPELLING PERFORMANCE IN PATIENTS I.G.R., J.G AND L.B.

The patterns of performance on word and nonword spelling tasks (spontaneous written narrative, written naming, oral and written spelling of words and nonwords) observed in the three patients considered in the present chapter are summarized in Table 2. It should be mentioned here that, although two patients (I.G.R. and L.B.) are native speakers of Italian and one patient (J.G.) is a native speaker of English, they have been submitted to tests which are largely comparable in structure. Both Italian and English patients were asked to spell list of words and nonwords. Word stimuli were controlled for frequency, grammatical class, orthographic 'regularity',[3] abstractness/concreteness and length. Nonword stimuli were controlled for length, degree of similarity to words and morphological decomposability (that is, the possibility to parse the stimulus nonword into nonpermissible sequences of roots and affixes).

The comparison of the results obtained in spelling tasks reveals important differences as regards the constellation of spared and impaired performance in patients I.G.R., J.G. and L.B.

The spontaneous written narratives produced by patient I.G.R. (Caramazza *et al.*, 1986) were error-free, as was his written naming. The patient wrote incorrectly to dictation only 17/628 familiar words (2.7%), but as many as 149/514 novel words (29%). It must be noted that the incidence of incorrect responses on nonword spelling tasks in normal Italian spellers, matched to I.G.R. for age and educational level, never exceeds 8%. Oral spelling was attempted with I.G.R., but he refused to cooperate, as he found the task extremely strange. The patient's reaction is not surprising. Since Italian is an orthographically "transparent" language (but see note 3), oral spelling is not taught at school and is not practised in adult life.

The spontaneous written narratives produced by patient J.G. (Goodman and Caramazza, 1986a), as well as her written description of the Cookie

TABLE 2

Comparison of the spelling performance obtained by patients I.G.R., J.G. and L.B.: incidence of errors in the various spelling tasks (percentages are in parentheses).

	I.G.R.	J.G.	L.B.
Spontaneous writing	Normal	Impaired	Impaired
Written naming	0/60 (0)	7/51 (14)	65/124 (52)
Written spelling to dictation:			
(a) Words	17/628 (3)	114/326 (35)	305/743 (41)
(b) Nonwords	149/514 (29)	34/34 (0)	246/425 (68)
Oral spelling to dictation:			
(a) Words		74/292 (25)	44/64 (69)
(b) Nonwords	—	33/34 (3)	49/64 (77)

Theft, were replete with spelling errors. In written naming she made 7 errors out of 51 stimuli (13.7%). In tasks requiring written spelling-to-dictation, J.G. wrote incorrectly 114/326 words (35%), but flawlessly wrote 34/34 nonwords. In oral spelling to dictation, the patient produced incorrect responses to 74/292 words (25.3%), but to only 1/34 nonwords (3%).

Patient L.B. (Caramazza *et al.*, 1987) produced syntactically and lexically sophisticated written narratives, marred by very frequent spelling errors. Written naming was severely impaired, as 65 spelling errors out of 124 responses to stimulus pictures were noted (52%). Written spelling to dictation was severely impaired for both words (305 incorrect responses out of 743 stimuli, 41%) and nonwords (246 incorrect responses out of 425 stimuli, 58%). Oral spelling to dictation was also severely impaired, as L.B. produced incorrect responses to 44/64 words (69%) and 49/64 nonwords (77%).

Even on a first pass, it is apparent that our subjects differ under important respects: I.G.R. shows normal word writing and impaired nonword writing; J.G. shows the opposite pattern: normal nonword spelling and poor word spelling (both oral and written); L.B. demonstrates a severe impairment of both word and nonword spelling (both oral and written). Thus, it must be tentatively, but confidently, concluded that the three patients are affected by damage to distinct components of the spelling process. The functional locus of lesion must now be identified in each patient.

3. ON LOCATING THE FUNCTIONAL LESION IN PATIENTS I.G.R., J.G. AND L.B.

The task of identifying the functional lesion(s) responsible for the spelling disorder observed in patients I.G.R., J.G. and L.B. is guided by considerations on the functional architecture of the spelling system, in the light of the observed patterns of spared and impaired performance.

3.1. *Patient I.G.R.: A Phonological Buffer Deficit*

The essentially flawless performance obtained by I.G.R. in tasks that require the ability to write words contrasts with his difficulty in nonword writing, and unequivocally points to the disruption of a component of the system involved in nonword writing, but not in word writing. Since phonological input processing is normal in this patient (he performs well within the normal range in tasks of phoneme discrimination and of auditory-visual matching that use minimal pairs of occlusive consonants embedded in CV syllables), damage must involve an output locus. Two output components required for nonword writing are present in the model sketched in Figure 1: the Phonological Buffer and the Phoneme-to-Grapheme Conversion system. The decision regarding the locus of lesion can be made on the basis of further information on the pattern of spared and impaired performance, and on the qualitative aspects of I.G.R.'s errors.

The Phonological Buffer and the Phoneme-to-Grapheme Conversion system differ under one important respect as regards their location in the general architecture of the cognitive system. The Phonological Buffer plays a crucial role in any tasks that require a phonological string to be stored in preparation for later processes. Hence, this component is necessary not only for nonword writing, but also for nonword reading and nonword repetition. By contrast, the Phoneme-to-Grapheme Conversion system is required only for nonword writing. The two components are also play a critically different role in the process of nonword writing: the Phonological Buffer is a short-term memory system, which holds a phonological nonword sequence as long as necessary for the string to be converted into an orthographic nonword sequence; the Phoneme-to-Grapheme Conversion system is a computational unit, responsible for the sequential mapping of the sequence of phonological segments stored in the Phonological Buffer onto an orthographic representation. On these premises, distinct patterns of deficit can be predicted as the result of damage to these two components of the spelling system. If I.G.R.'s lesion is at the level of the Phonological Buffer, an association of symptoms is expected: writing, reading and repetition of nonwords should all be disrupted to a comparable degree. Furthermore, the same error type(s) should be observed across tasks; and the nature of the errors must be compatible with the disruption of the procedures normally performed by the buffer. If the patient's functional lesion disrupts the Phoneme-to-Grapheme Conversion system, only nonword writing should be impaired, and difficulties in nonword reading and repetition, if present at all, should be accounted for by damage to independent components — i.e., the stimulus—error relationship in these two tasks should be different from that observed in nonword writing.

I.G.R. was submitted to nonword reading and nonword repetition tasks. Some examples of errors made by the patient in nonword writing, reading and repetition are reported in Table 3. The results obtained by I.G.R. in the three tasks, displayed for comparison in Tables 4—6, are compatible with the hypothesis of damage to the Phonological Buffer, but not with the hypothesis of damage to the Phoneme-to-Grapheme Conversion system. The figures reported in Table 4 demonstrate that nonword writing, reading and repetition are impaired to a comparable extent. As expected from the fact that a non-lexical component is disrupted, only 3/149 errors in nonword writing (2%), 9/78 errors in reading (11.5%) and1/103 errors in repetition (1%) are words. More important, the same error types are

TABLE 3

Patient I.G.R.: Examples of phonologically related errors made in writing to dictation, reading and repetition of novel words.

(a) *Writing*

efile → evile	cecchio → cechio
birdi → birti	dochio → docchio
uttico → uttito	

(b) *Reading*

diffa → biffa	arrasti → arasti (you sowed)
elvitare → elvidare	ripano → rippano
trefova → trevova	

(c) *Repetition*

tacro → tagro	sganutta → sganuta
brasna → crasna	metinace → metinacce
telpito → telpido	

TABLE 4

Patient I.G.R.: Incidence of errors in writing, reading and repetition of nonwords.

Writing	149/514	(29.0%)
Reading	78/505	(15.5%)
Repetition	103/426	(24.2%)
Total	330/1445	(22.8%)

observed across tasks (Table 5). A very high (and comparable across tasks) percentage of errors consists of the substitution, insertion, deletion or transposition of a single phoneme/grapheme of the stimulus (76.5% in writing, 83.4% in reading, 60.5% in repetition). Also the combined incidence of multiple errors, consisting of more than one substitution or insertion or deletion error in the same response, and of mixed errors, consisting of one or more occurrences of at least two error types, is comparable across tasks (multiple + mixed errors: 18.1% in writing, 16.7% in reading, 18.3% in repetition). The similarity observed in the semi-qualitative error analysis just reported emerges even more clearly when a finer-grained analysis is performed, in an attempt at defining a principled stimulus—error relationship. In all tasks, the incorrect responses produced by I.G.R. are for the most part phonologically related to the stimulus, that is, the graphemes (in writing) and the phonemes (in reading and repetition) produced incorrectly share manner of articulation

GABRIELE MICELI

TABLE 5

Patient I.G.R.: Analysis of the errors made in writing to dictation, reading and repeating nonwords (percentages are in parentheses).

	Writing	Reading	Repetition
Single-letter errors			
Substitutions	78 (52.3)	57 (67.9)	51 (49.0)
Insertions	15 (10.1)	9 (10.7)	7 (6.7)
Deletions	19 (12.8)	4 (4.8)	2 (1.9)
Transpositions	2 (1.3)		3 (2.9)
Multiple-letter errors			
Multiple Subst.	15 (10.1)	8 (9.5)	15 (14.4)
Multiple Insert.	1 (0.7)		1 (1.0)
Multiple Delet.		1 (1.2)	
Subst. + Insert.	3 (2.0)	4 (4.8)	2 (1.9)
Subst. + Delet.	2 (1.3)		1 (1.0)
Subst. + Transp.		1 (1.2)	
Delet. + Insert.	2 (1.3)		
Delet. + Transp.	3 (2.0)		
Sub. + Delet. + Transp.	1 (0.7)		
Stress	1 (0.7)		
Neologism	1 (0.7)		
Fragments	6 (4.0)		22 (21.2)
Total	149 (100)	84 (100)	104 (100)

TABLE 6

Patient I.G.R.: Incidence of incorrect responses in nonword writing, reading and repetition as a function of stimulus length.

	Stimulus length (in letters)		
	4—5	6—7	8—9
Writing	19.5	26.4	38.1
Reading	12.2	18.0	14.8
Repetition	10.4	21.5	32.9

(e.g., occlusives, fricatives, liquids, etc.) with the target graphemes/phonemes, but differ as for voicing (voiced vs. voiceless) and/or place of articulation (e.g., bilabial, alveolar, velar, etc.). On nonword tasks, phonologically related responses account for 122/130 errors in writing (93.8%), for 67/83 errors in reading (80.7%) and for 85/104 errors in repetition (82%). Also compatible with the Phonological Buffer damage hypothesis is the observation of a length effect in nonword writing and repetition (Table 6). The absence of a length effect in nonword reading can be explained with task-specific requirements: in writing and repetition the to-be-written nonword is presented as a fleeting auditory stimulus, whereas in reading the stimulus is presented visually, and remains in view long enough for the patient to make repeated attempts at producing the correct response.

To sum up, the normal performance in word writing, the association of poor writing, reading and repetition of nonwords, the comparable incidence of phonologically related errors in all impaired tasks and the length effect in the tasks that use auditory input converge in indicating the Phonological Buffer as the locus of lesion in patient, I.G.R.[4]

3.2. *Patient J.G.: A Graphemic Output Lexicon Deficit*

The most striking feature observed in J.G.'s case is the superior performance in nonword spelling with respect to word spelling. This pattern can only result from an impairment of the lexical procedures responsible for word writing. Since the results of comprehension tasks demonstrate that J.G. is able to understand auditorily presented words, the only possible locus of lesion is the Graphemic Output Lexicon. This hypothesis can be evaluated by matching the predictions made on the basis of the putative role assigned to the Graphemic Output Lexicon in the proposed model with the pattern of results obtained by J.G. in various spelling tasks.

If the unavailability of orthographic word entries in the Graphemic Output Lexicon is responsible for the observed disorder, spelling performance should be affected by lexical variables. Also, more specific predictions can be made regarding the nature of the incorrect responses expected in the case of J.G. According to the model of spelling sketched in Figure 1, the unavailability of lexical entries should force the patient to produce a (written or oral) spelling response through phonological mediation. As a consequence, the misspellings produced in response to items that are not available in the Graphemic Output Lexicon should reflect the operation of Phoneme-to-Grapheme Conversion mechanisms. The incorrect responses produced in all word spelling tasks by J.G. should result from the application of graphemic options that are legal in English, but are inappropriate for the specific lexical entry that the patient is asked to spell. Thus, as in other patients with lexical damage reported in the literature (e.g., Beauvois and Dérouesné, 1981; Hatfield and Patterson, 1983; Goodman and Caramazza, 1986b), the errors produced by J.G. should be for the most part phonologically plausible, and should be nonwords (e.g., coarse → koarse).

The pattern of performance observed in J.G. is clearly consistent with damage to the Graphemic Output Lexicon. All the errors in written naming (7/51, 13.7%) were produced to stimuli in the mid- to low-frequency range. High-frequency words were spelled with significantly fewer errors than low-frequency items (errors in written spelling: high-frequency: 22/146, 15% vs. low-frequency: 79/146, 54%; errors in oral spelling: high-frequency: 16/146, 11% vs. 58/146, 40%). Orthographic "regularity" affected J.G.'s performance, "regular" words being spelled more accurately than "irregular" words. No effects of grammatical class, abstractness/concreteness and length were observed. Some examples of the errors produced by J.G. in oral and written spelling are reported in Table 7. As it can be seen, these errors are all phonologically plausible: writing /goulz/ as 'goles' instead of 'goals' results from incorrectly converting the phonological segment /ou/ into the graphemic option 'o' instead of 'oa', and the phonological sequence /lz/ into 'les' instead of 'ls'; writing /bitreid/ as 'betrade' instead of 'betrayed' derives from choosing for the sequence /eid/ the incorrect option 'ade' instead of 'ayed', which is appropriate for the target word; and so on.

Thus, it can be confidently concluded that the cognitive locus of damage in patient J.G., as in other patients described in the literature (Beauvois and Dérouesné, 1981; Hatfield and Patterson, 1983; Goodman and Caramazza, 1986b), is the Graphemic Output Lexicon. The phonologically plausible, incorrect responses produced by the patient result from attempts at spelling by using the Phoneme-to-Grapheme Conversion system.

TABLE 7

Patient J.G.: Examples of phonologically plausible errors produced in spelling words to dictation.

(a) Written spelling	(b) Oral spelling
ruin → rewin	beak → beek
halo → haylow	yawn → yon
goals → goles	rigid → ridgid
injure → enjor	igloo → iglu
betrayed → betrade	basis → basess
curtain → kirtin	caught → cought
ultimate → altimit	length → lenth
nuisance → newcence	status → stattice
negotiate → negosheate	certain → sertin
suggesting → cidgesting	chipmunk → cheepmonk

3.3. *Patient L.B.: A Graphemic Buffer Deficit*

The quantitative results displayed in Table 2 indicate that, contrary to

I.G.R. (selective impairment of nonword writing) and J.G. (selective impairment of word spelling), both word and nonword spelling are impaired in the case of L.B., in the written and in the oral modality.

L.B.'s deficit in spelling cannot result from some input disorder, as the patient shows poor performance in all spelling tasks (spontaneous writing, written naming, oral and written spelling-to-dictation, delayed copy), independent of input modality, and shows normal processing of auditory input. Thus, the disorder in this patient must be located at an output locus which, when lesioned, results in poor oral and written spelling of both familiar and novel words. In the context of the proposed model, the pattern of errors observed in L.B. admits to two alternative explanations.

In the first place, L.B.'s pattern of performance might result from a deficit that affects two independent components, one normally used for word spelling (i.e., the Graphemic Output Lexicon), the other normally used for nonword spelling (i.e., the Phonological Output Lexicon or the Phoneme-to-Grapheme Conversion system). Alternatively, the observed performance might result from damage to only one component, used in oral and written spelling of both words and nonwords (i.e., the Grapheme Buffer). The putative architecture of the spelling system predicts distinct patterns of impairment for the two hypotheses. If independent damage to lexical and phonological mechanisms is responsible for L.B.'s disorder, performance accuracy in word and nonword tasks should be sensitive to distinct factors and the types of errors in word and nonword spelling should also differ. In particular, word spelling should be sensitive to lexical variables; and the performance in nonword spelling should be compatible with damage to the Phonological Buffer or to the Phoneme-to-Grapheme Conversion system (these patterns of errors have been described in the paragraph discussing the performance of patient I.G.R.). If L.B.'s poor spelling results from damage to only one component, errors on words and nonwords should be quantitatively comparable and qualitatively of the same type(s). A much more detailed analysis of L.B.'s performance in spelling and spelling-related tasks than reported so far is necessary in order to decide between the double-deficit and the single-deficit hypothesis.

A summary of L.B.'s performance in various spelling tasks is presented in Table 8. All spelling tasks are severely impaired, with the exception of the direct copy of words and nonwords. L.B. wrote to dictation high-frequency and low-frequency words with the same accuracy, independent of abstractness/concreteness, grammatical class and orthographic "regularity" (see note 3). In nonword writing, no effects of similarity to words and of morphological structure were observed. In both word and nonword spelling, only stimulus length systematically affected performance accuracy. The effect of length in word and nonword writing-to-dictation tasks is presented as an example in Table 9. In addition, L.B. flawlessly

TABLE 8

Patient L.B.: Summary of the performance obtained in the various spelling tasks (percentages in parentheses).

	Words	Nonwords
Written spelling-to-dictation	305/743 (41)	246/425 (58)
Oral spelling-to-dictation	44/64 (69)	49/64 (77)
Written naming	65/124 (52)	
Copy from a model	5/57 (9)	2/56 (4)
Delayed copy	21/59 (36)	38/60 (63)

TABLE 9

Patient L.B.: Length effect in writing words and nonwords to dictation (percentages in parentheses).

Stimulus length	Words	Nonwords
4—5	37/242 (15)	31/113 (27)
6—7	90/264 (34)	79/155 (51)
8—9	100/150 (67)	64/85 (75)
10—12	78/87 (90)	74/74 (100)
Total	305/743 (41)	246/425 (58)

wrote to dictation 100 meaningless CV syllables. His incorrect responses were for the most part orthographically similar to the stimulus, but they were not phonologically plausible, nor phonologically related (a more detailed analysis of L.B.'s spelling errors is reported below). The reading performance of this patient has been extensively analysed in Caramazza *et al.* (1985) and will not be considered at length here. L.B. displayed essentially normal word reading (8 errors out of 388 stimuli, 2%), and very poor reading of nonwords which could not be decomposed into morphological segments (95 errors out of 180 stimuli, 52.8%). Errors in reading were not of the phonologically related type. In repetition, L.B. produced correct responses to 72/72 words, but made 3 errors to 72 nonwords (4.2%). Also in this task, errors were phonologically unrelated.

These results do not support the 'double deficit' hypothesis. The lack of sensitivity to lexical factors and the absence of phonologically plausible spelling errors rules out damage to the Graphemic Output Lexicon. Also the possibility that L.B.'s deficit in nonword spelling results from damage to the Phonological Buffer or to the Phoneme-to-Grapheme Conversion system is disconfirmed by our results. Damage to the Phonological Buffer should result in comparable impairment of nonword writing, reading and repetition (see paragraph on patient I.G.R.). By contrast, L.B. shows a high incidence of errors in nonword writing (58%) and reading (52.8%), but a much lower incidence of errors in nonword repetition (4.2%). This pattern of performance and the observation that errors on nonwords in all tasks are for the most part phonologically unrelated rule out Phonological Buffer damage. The alternative possibility that damage to the Phoneme-to-Grapheme Conversion system is responsible for poor nonword writing is disconfirmed by L.B.'s error-free performance in CV-syllable writing. To sum up, consideration of the overall performance observed in this patient allows to exclude that his misspellings result from independent damage to lexical and phonological mechanisms.

Having ruled out alternative explanations, the single-deficit hypothesis that locates damage at the level of the Graphemic Buffer can now be entertained. Evaluation of this hypothesis must be guided by the role putatively assigned to this Buffer in the process of spelling. The Grapheme Buffer temporarily stores graphemic representations of words and nonwords alike, prior to their conversion into abstractly coded letters (for written spelling), letter names (for oral spelling) or hand/finger movements (for typing). As a consequence, the errors observed after damage to this buffer should be equally distributed across words and nonwords, both quantitatively and qualitatively. In addition, incorrect responses should reflect the loss of orthographic information on individual items stored in the buffer, or the loss of ordinal information attached to each item in the orthographic string. The data reported so far support the Graphemic Buffer deficit hypothesis, as indicated by the lack of lexical effects and the systematic length effect in word and nonword spelling, and by the observation that the spelling errors made by L.B. were not phonologically related (as in I.G.R., who has damage to the Phonological Buffer), nor phonologically plausible (as in J.G., who has damage to the Graphemic Output Lexicon and produces spelling responses by mapping sounds to graphemic options). In order to verify the Grapheme Buffer hypothesis more stringently, qualitative analyses were performed on the corpus of errors obtained from L.B.

The analysis reveals that the incorrect responses produced by the patient can be classified into substitutions, insertions, deletions or trans-positions of single or of multiple letters, into mixed errors (one or more occurrences of two or more error types) and into unclassifiable errors, in which no apparent relationship exists between stimulus and incorrect response. Examples of these error types are reported in Table 10. The distribution of these error types confirms that length is the critical factor that affects L.B.'s performance. Not only is the incidence of correct responses significantly lower on long than on short items, but the production of long items is more disrupted than the production of short items. As a matter of fact, in writing words to dictation, complex (mixed and unrelated) errors account for only 3/37 errors produced by L.B. on 4—5 letter stimuli (8.1%), but for as many as 55/78 incorrect responses produced to 10—12 letter words (60.5%).

One aspect of L.B.'s performance not fully compatible with the Grapheme Buffer hypothesis is the consistent superiority of word over nonword spelling. However, this quantitative difference is not sufficient to disconfirm the Grapheme Buffer damage hypothesis, since poorer performance in nonword writing as opposed to word writing could be explained by the subtle deficit observed in nonword repetition, or by some other deficit, not related to Grapheme Buffer damage. A further error analysis unequivocally confirms the hypothesis that L.B.'s disorder results from Grapheme Buffer damage. Since the buffer plays the same role in word and nonword writing, the incidence of substitution, insertion, deletion and transposition errors in word and nonword writing-to-dictation should be comparable. The incidence of these error types, displayed in Table 11, is identical across words and nonwords. Thus, the spelling

TABLE 10

Patient L.B.: Examples of the errors made in writing words and nonwords to dictation.

Words	Nonwords
(a) *Single errors*	
binario (track) → bilario	inatili → inavili
comincia (he begins) → cuomincia	ispi → inspi
incontra (he meets) → inconra	intarno → intano
maniglia (handle) → magnilia	bidegna → dibegna
(b) *Multiple errors*	
bagaglio (baggage) → bolaglio	signoge → signece
amerai (you will love) → amerirai	chierova → chiova
raccontare (to tell) → racconae	spizegia → spegia
(c) *Mixed errors*	
pensiero (thought) → periero	ondaso → adaso
pulizia (cleanliness) → puziala	fralte → flate
davanti (ahead) → danati	fracca → facra
furgone (van) prunone	stovidi → dosidi
(d) *Unrelated errors*	
finestra (window) → fesfera	fomigna → fugnona
personaggi (characters) → porsiongi	toglieri → terlele

disorder demonstrated by L.B. can be confidently attributed to a disorder of the Grapheme Buffer.[5]

TABLE 11
Patient L.B.: Incidence of single and multiple substitutions, insertions, deletions and transpositions in word and nonword writing-to-dictation (percentages in parentheses).

	Words	Nonwords
Substitutions	65 (37)	41 (36)
Insertions	14 (8)	10 (9)
Deletions	61 (34)	42 (37)
Transpositions	38 (21)	21 (18)
Total	178	114

To sum up, even though the spelling errors made by the three patients described here are very similar, the careful analysis of the patterns of spelling performance displayed by the three subjects allows to demonstrate that they result from damage to distinct components of the spelling system. Patient I.G.R. has damage to the Phonological Buffer. He writes words normally, but writes (and reads and repeats) nonwords poorly; the incidence of spelling errors in writing and repetition is a function of stimulus length; most incorrect responses are phonologically related to the stimulus. Patient J.G. has damage to the Graphemic Output Lexicon. She spells nonwords flawlessly, but makes many errors in word spelling. The incidence of errors in these tasks is a function of stimulus frequency and of orthographic regularity; most incorrect responses are phonologically plausible, and result from the lexically unconstrained use of the Phoneme-to-Grapheme Conversion system. Patient L.B. has damage to the Grapheme Buffer. He spells both words and nonwords very poorly. His performance is unaffected by lexical variables, but is sensitive to stimulus length. The same error types are observed (with an extremely similar incidence) in word and nonword spelling.

4. DISCUSSION

For a long time, research on dysgraphia has focused on proposing taxonomies, based either on the anatomo-clinical correlates of the disorder (e.g., Benson, 1979) or on the symptom-complexes observed in dysgraphic patients (e.g., Hécaen and Albert, 1978). In recent years, investigations in the cognitive neuropsychology of spelling have been concerned with issues regarding the functional architecture of this process, both in normality and in pathology (for a review, see Ellis, 1982 and 1989; Margolin, 1984; Miceli, 1989; Patterson, 1989). As the result of these studies, an articulated model of spelling has been proposed, which has received support from both theoretical considerations and empirical evidence. The functional architecture of the present version of the model serves as a guideline for current investigations, the goal of which is the formulation of updated (that is, computationally more explicit) versions of the model.

The theoretical background provided by a computationally explicit model is something that research on spelling cannot do without, independent of whether the aim of a study is the understanding of the normal system or the theoretically defensible characterization of spelling disorders. A first goal of the present investigation was to demonstrate that, beyond apparent similarities, variations could be revealed in the pattern of impairment observed in three dysgraphic patients. A more important goal of this study was to verify that it is possible to make motivated decisions as to whether across-patients variations merely result from quantitative differences or from damage to distinct components of the cognitive system. Without a theory of normal cognitive abilities, either it would be impossible to make any decisions, or the decision would have to be based entirely on intuitive criteria. Within a cognitive model, a principled analysis allows motivated decisions. The functional architecture of the model establishes on theoretically defensible grounds the set of observations over which the patients' performance must be evaluated. Explicit hypotheses on the overall pattern of performance and on the types of errors that are expected as the result of damage to each component of the normal system can be formulated. The performance predicted on the basis of theoretical considerations can thus be matched with the observed performance. Only this type of analysis makes it possible to interpret across-patient variations properly.

The empirical results reported in the present chapter confirm the metatheoretical claim (Caramazza, 1986) that a computationally explicit model is the necessary prerequisite for theoretically driven analyses of pathological behavior. One current cognitive model of the spelling process has been used here in order to guide the investigation of the performance obtained by three cognitively impaired subjects, whose spelling errors were apparently similar. The model led to make detailed predictions on the disorders that were expected as the result of damage to various components of the system. The analysis of the data, guided by these theoretical considerations, allowed to demonstrate that the differences observed among the three patients, resulted from damage to distinct components of the spelling system.

NOTES

[1] This research was supported in part by NIH grant NS 22201 and by a grant from the Ministro della Sanità. I also wish to thank Roberta Ann Goodman and Alfonso Caramazza for making available the corpus of errors produced by patient J.G.

[2] That is, patients classified as exemplars of a category according to clinical criteria are indeed considered as possibly cognitively heterogeneous, but it is assumed that the amount of within-category variation is lesser than the amount of across-category variation.

[3] Italian and English differ greatly as regards the "transparency" of sound-to-print mappings. English is a highly "opaque" language, where as a rule the same phonological segment corresponds to several graphemic options, and where many words have totally idiosyncratic spellings (e.g., /yɔt/ → yacht). By contrast, Italian is an almost entirely "transparent" language. There are no words with truly "irregular" spelling, and sound-to-print correspondences are usually unambiguous. Some exceptions are present, though. Some mappings between phonemes and graphemes are ambiguous, since some (albeit very few) phonological segments admit to two graphemic options. Hence, there is a small number of words in the language whose orthography cannot be predicted by phonology, and is uniquely specified only at the lexical level. Thus, for example, the phonological segment /kwɔ/ corresponds to two different graphemic options — compare /kwɔko/ → cuoco (the cook) and /kwɔta/ → quota (the quote), respectively. A list consisting of words with ambiguous phoneme-to-grapheme correspondences was thus administered to the Italian patients.

It must be noted that the terms "regularity" and "transparency" are used here to denote an intuitive notion, that is, the predictability of the orthography of a word from its phonology. For a principled analysis of "regularity" and "transparency" in terms of the probability of occurrence of the phoneme-to-grapheme correspondences present in a particular word, see Goodman and Caramazza (1986b).

[4] It must be mentioned here that although, as we have said, I.G.R. refused to perform oral spelling tasks, the functional architecture of the spelling system leads to predict his performance straightforwardly: in the case of damage to the Phonological Buffer, word spelling should be unimpaired, but nonword spelling should be poor. In addition, as in written nonword spelling, errors in oral spelling should be more frequently produced in response to short as opposed to long items, and should be phonologically related to the stimulus.

[5] For a further analysis of the spelling disorder in this patient, see Caramazza and Miceli (in press).

REFERENCES

Beauvois, M. F. and Dérouesné, J.: 1981, 'Lexical or orthographic agraphia', *Brain* **104**, 21—49.

Benson, F. D.: 1979, *Aphasia, Alexia and Agraphia*, Churchill Livingston, New York.

Campbell, R.: 1983, 'Writing nonwords to dictation', *Brain and Language* **19**, 153—178.

Caramazza, A.: 1986, 'On drawing inferences about the structure of normal cognitive systems from the analysis of patterns of impaired performance: The case for single-patient studies', *Brain and Cognition* **5**, 41—66.

Caramazza, A. and Badecker, W.: 1989, 'Patient classification in neuropsychological research', *Brain and Cognition* **10**, 256—295.

Caramazza, A. and Mc Closkey, 1988, 'The case for single patient studies', *Cognitive Neuropsychology* **5**, 517—528.

Caramazza, A. and Miceli, G.: (in press), 'The structure of orthographic representations'. *Cognition*.

Caramazza, A., Miceli, G., Silveri, M. C. and Laudanna, A.: 1985, 'Reading mechanisms and the organization of the lexicon: Evidence from acquired dyslexia', *Cognitive Neuropsychology* **2**, 81—114.

Caramazza, A., Miceli, G. and Villa, G.: 1986, 'The role of the (Output) Phonological Buffer in reading, writing and repetition', *Cognitive Neuropsychology* **3**, 37—76.

Caramazza, A., Miceli, G., Villa, G. and Romani, C.: 1987, 'The role of the Graphemic Buffer in spelling: Evidence from a case of acquired dysgraphia', *Cognition* **26**, 59—85.

Ellis, A. W.: 1982, 'Spelling and writing (and reading and speaking)', in A. W. Ellis (ed.), *Normality and Pathology in Cognitive Functions*, Academic Press, London.

Ellis, A. W. (in press) 'Modeling the spelling process', in G. Denes, C. Sementa, P. Biziacchi and E. Andreewski (eds.) *Perspectives in Cognitive Neuropsychology*. Lawrence Erlbaum association, Hillsdale, NY.

Glushko, R. J.: 1981, 'Principles of pronouncing print: The psychology of phonography', in A. M. Lesgold and C. A. Perfetti (eds.), *Interactive Processes in Reading*, Lawrence Erlbaum Associates, Hillsdale, NJ.

Goodman, R. A. and Caramazza, A.: 1986a, 'Aspects of the spelling process: Evidence from a case of acquired dysgraphia', *Language and Cognitive Processes* **1**, 263—296.

Goodman, R. A. and Caramazza, A.: 1986b, 'Dissociation of spelling errors in written and oral spelling: The role of allographic conversion in writing', *Cognitive Neuropsychology* **3**, 179—206.

Hatfield, F. M. and Patterson, K. E.: 1983, 'Phonological spelling', *Quarterly Journal of Experimental Psychology* **35A**, 451—468.

Hécaen, H. and Albert, M. A.: 1978, *Human Neuropsychology*, Wiley, New York.

Henderson, L.: 1982, *Orthographies and Reading*, Lawrence Erlbaum Associates, Hillsdale, NJ.

Kay, J. and Marcel, T.: 1981, 'One process, not two, in reading aloud: Lexical analogies do the work of non-lexical rules', *Quarterly Journal of Experimental Psychology* **33A**, 397—413.

Marcel, T.: 1980, 'Surface dyslexia and beginning reading: A revised hypothesis of the pronunciation of print and its impairment', in M. Coltheart, K. E. Patterson and J. C. Marshall (eds.) *Deep Dyslexia*, Routledge and Kegan Paul, London.

Margolin, D. I.: 1984, 'The neuropsychology of writing and spelling: Semantic, phonological, motor, and perceptual processes', *Quarterly Journal of Experimental Psychology* **36A**, 459—489.

Miceli, G.: 1989, 'A cognitive model of spelling: Evidence from cognitively-impaired subjects', in P. G. Aaron and R. Malatesha Joshi (eds.), Reading and Writing disorders in different orthographic systems. Kluwer Academic Publishers, Dordrecht, The Netherlands.

Miceli, G., Silveri, M. C., Romani, C. and Caramazza, A.: 1989, 'Variation in the pattern of omission of grammatical markers in so-called agrammatic patients', *Brain and Language* **36**, 447—492.

Patterson, K. E.: 1989, 'Acquired disorders of spelling', in G. Denes, C. Semenza, P. Bisiacchi and E. Andreewski (eds.), *Perspectives in Cognitive Neuropsychology*. Lawrence Erlbaum Associates, Hillsdale, NJ.

Shallice, T.: 1981, 'Phonological agraphia and the lexical route in writing', *Brain* **104**, 413—429.

YVAN LEBRUN AND LUC DE VREESE

PURE ALEXIA

1. INTRODUCTION

In 1906 the French neurologist Pierre Marie published two papers on aphasia which caused much commotion in neurological circles, because they advocated a complete revision of classical views on aphasia. One of the concepts which Marie proposed to discard was the notion of selective impairment of only one verbal modality. Thus, he rejected the idea that there could be anything like pure word deafness, i.e., a selective disorder of speech comprehension.

While he denied the existence of a disturbance affecting exclusively the comprehension of speech, Marie conceded that a number of patients exhibited an impairment that showed almost exclusively in reading (Figure 1). For instance, in his second paper on the revision of classical aphasiological views, he stated that, in contradistinction to pure word deafness which did not really exist, pure word blindness was an actual nosological entity.

Ever since, the existence of an acquired selective impairment of reading has generally been admitted. The disorder has been given various names, such as "pure alexia", "optic alexia", "agnosic alexia", "alexia without agraphia" and, more recently, "alexia resulting from a visuo-verbal disconnection". Since it implies no etiological explanation, the descriptive label "pure alexia" will be used here.

Many reports of pure alexia are to be found in the literature. From them it is possible to cull the symptomatology of the condition, which appears to show a number of variations.

2. SYMPTOMATOLOGY

2.1. *Reading Difficulties*

The cardinal symptom of pure alexia is a marked reading disorder which stands out in contrast to the relative preservation of the other verbal modalities. In particular, there is no gross aphasia and written expression remains possible.

The reading impairment is not uniform. On the contrary, there are considerable inter-individual differences as regards the severity of the disturbance, the kind of material which is difficult to decipher, and the concomitant symptoms.

R. M. Joshi (ed.), Written Language Disorders, 105–126.
© 1991 *Kluwer Academic Publishers. Printed in the Netherlands.*

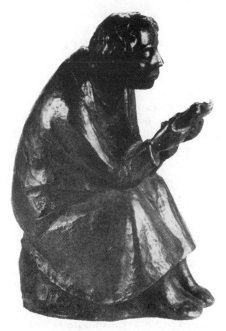

Fig. 1. Reading.

2.1.1. *Global Alexia*

Some patients can read neither words nor individual letters. Their alexia is global.

Despite their inability to identify individual letters and to understand written words, global alexics generally can match letters or written words. They perform well on such a matching task because it does not imply recognition of the stimuli.

At times, partial recognition is achieved, however, as when the patient manages to distinguish between letters which are correctly positioned and letters which are presented upside down or sideways.

Pure alexia is not always global. A number of patients can easily identify some components of written language or can identify some components more readily than others. For instance, there are alexics who have less difficulty in recognizing letters than words. Their alexia is primarily verbal. Conversely, words may be less hard to identify than letters, in which case the alexia is said to be primarily literal. Some authors refer to verbal alexia as "word blindness", and to literal alexia as "letter blindness".

2.1.2 *Literal Alexia*

When patients have difficulty in reading letters, the difficulty may vary with the way the letters are presented. For instance, the patient of Stachowiak and Poeck (1976) gave 70% correct answers when he had to name letters presented one at a time, but his score dropped to 30% when he had to name letters in words. On the contrary, a patient of ours gave 80% correct answers when he had to name isolated letters. His score rose to 91% when the letters were presented in words.

A number of errors made by patients when identifying letters can be classified as morphological or graphic: they are confusions of letters which resemble each other, e.g., "A" and "H", or are mirror-images, e.g., "b" and "d". Other errors are phonic: the names of the letters which are confused resemble one another, e.g., "s" and "f". At times, however, there appears to be no morphological and no phonic relationship between stimulus and response.

When identifying series of letters, some patients tend to give the same response several times in succession. They perseverate. It is often unclear whether they cannot help repeating the previous response (efferent perseveration) or whether they think they are shown the same letter several times (afferent perseveration).

2.1.3. *Static Alexia*

Some literal alexics have less difficulty in reading letters when these are drawn in front of them, that is to say when they can watch them being produced. Such patients are said to have primarily "static alexia". For instance, a patient of Botez *et al.*, (1964) could read letters drawn with a lighted cigarette in a dark room better than letters of the same size presented to him on sheets of paper.

Occasionally, the patient can read better if the sheet of paper with the letter on it is slowly moved in front of him.

2.1.4. *Nonvisual Identification of Letters*

Patients who find it difficult to identify letters by sight may be able to recognize them fairly easily if they trace them with their finger or if they reproduce them with their finger in the air. This reading through kinesthesia is known as "Wilbrand's manoeuver". Contrary to Dejerine's assumption (1892) not every pure alexic can successfully use arthrokinesia to identify letters, as the cases reported by Beringer and Stein (1930) and by Ombredane (1944) show.

When patients are able to copy, they may resort to writing to identify letters. For instance, the patient of Dünsing (1953a) used to write the letters she could not recognize by sight. Generally, once she had produced the letter herself, she was able to name it.

Tactile recognition of three-dimensional letters may be preserved in pure alexia, as the case reported by Stachowiak and Poeck (1976) shows.

Not infrequently dermolexia (also called "graphesthesia"), i.e., the ability to recognize letters drawn on the skin, is intact (e.g., Vincent *et al.*, 1977). In the case reported by Lhermitte and Beauvois (1973), on the contrary, it was severely disturbed.

When assessing dermolexia or the ability to identify three- dimensional letters, one should beware of a possible reduction of sensitivity in the right hand. Poor identification of the tactile stimulus may simply be a consequence of the hypesthesia. Bilateral testing is therefore desirable.

2.1.5. *Distinguishing between Letters and Nonletters*

A number of patients with literal alexia can distinguish letters from other graphic signs, even though they fail to identify the individual letters correctly (e.g., Assal and Zander, 1975). Often, as in the third case reported by Lebrun *et al.*, (1979), they are able to discriminate between letters they are familiar with (e.g., letters from the Latin alphabet) and foreign letters (e.g., Cyrillic characters).

2.1.6. *Verbal Alexia*

Some patients find the reading of words more difficult than the reading of individual letters. For instance, Stachowiak and Poeck's patient (1976), while unable to read words, was 70% of the time correct when he had to identify isolated letters. The patient of Ajax *et al.*, (1977) could generally identify isolated letters but found the reading of monosyllables difficult and the reading of polysyllabic words impossible.

On the whole, long or unfamiliar words are more troublesome than short and familiar ones. For instance, the second patient of Lebrun *et al.*, (1979) found the reading of French articles, prepositions and pronouns, most of which are monosyllabic, easier than the reading of content words having three or four syllables. However, as in the case reported by Beringer and Stein (1930), short function words may prove more difficult to identify than longer content words.

Although his alexia was nearly total, Dejerine's patient (1892) could generally recognize his name, whether presented alone or in a series of words. And Dejerine and Pelissier's first patient (1914) could recognize his name, and tell when it had been misspelled, although he could not correct the error.

The reading errors of verbal alexics can usually be divided into morphological paralexias (also called, though less appropriately, "visual errors") and semantic paralexias. For instance, on one occasion, the patient of Warrington and Zangwill (1957) misread "breaking" as "breakfast", and "months" as "weeks". The French-speaking patient of Lebrun and Devreux (1984) misread "carotte" (= carrot) as "cacao", and "Venice" as "Salzburg".

Typically, the patient with pure alexia is uncertain of his responses. Most of the time he gives hesitant answers and can easily be persuaded that he has misread the stimulus, even if he, in fact, has read it correctly.

At times, the patient's response shows that he has been able to access the semantic field to which the word to be read belongs but he cannot identify the word more specifically. For instance, the patient of Beringer and Stein (1930) once misread the German word "Indien" (= India) as "Elefant" (= elephant). She spontaneously commented that she had immediately recognized that the stimulus was a foreign word, that it evoked something which was far away, in the tropics. Then she came to think of elephants. She added that she had always liked elephants.

Patients may be able to distinguish between foreign words and words belonging to their mother-tongue even though they cannot read them (as in the case reported by Pillon et al., 1987).

No pure alexic seems to have ever been reported who could not recognize written language for what it was. Even when he is totally unable to read, the patient knows that he is looking at letters or at written words. Pure alexia, then, is not agnosia for written language, i.e., failure to recognize the nature of written language. Rather, it is agnosia for the symbolic value of the components of written language.

2.1.7. So-called Spelling Dyslexia

Patients who can read letters more easily than words sometimes use a stratagem to read words: they identify one by one the letters forming the word to be read and then mentally synthesize the word. This deciphering technique is often called "spelling dyslexia".

When the word is relatively long, patients may identify the first few letters and then guess at the rest. For instance, the third patient of Lebrun et al., (1979), when shown the French word "parapluie" (= umbrella), painfully identified the first two letters and then said: "Paraffine".

Occasionally, patients are encountered who can easily identify the letters forming the words they are shown, but prove unable to synthesize the words from the identified letters, possibly as a consequence of an impairment of short-term memory. Dide and Botcazo reported such a case in 1902.

2.1.8. Arthrokinesia

Some patients resort to arthrokinesia to read the words they cannot identify by sight. For instance, a patient of Botez and Serbanescu (1967), when she could not read a word, would reproduce it with her finger in her palm. This trick generally enabled her to identify the word.

2.1.9. *Factors Influencing the Reading Performance*

Usually, pure alexics find the reading of script more difficult than the reading of print. However, occasionally patients are encountered to whom it makes no difference (as in Dejerine's case, 1892).

When the system of writing comprises two types of signs, the reading difficulty may present differently according to the type to be deciphered. For instance, Sasanuma's patient (1974) could read kana symbols only by following their contours with his finger (Wildbrand's manoeuvre). Once the syllabic components had been identified in this way he could synthesize the word. On the other hand, kanji symbols were either identified swiftly by sight or not identified at all. Tracing their strokes with the finger did not help. Moreover, compound ideograms proved to be not more difficult to identify than simple ones.

If the patient is conversant with several languages, reading may not be affected to the same degree in each of them. For instance, an English patient of Hinshelwood (1902) had far less difficulty in reading Greek, and less difficulty in reading Latin and French, than in reading his mother-tongue.

Reading may be considerably better if the patient knows to what semantic field the words to be read belong. For instance, the reading performances of the patient of Beringer and Stein (1930) improved dramatically when she was told the semantic category to which the words to be read belonged. As for the patient of Pillon *et al.* (1987), he could not pick out the odd word in a series of three if he knew nothing about these words. But, if he was told that one of the words denoted an animal, or a fruit, or a profession, he could find it. Linguistic cuing then may facilitate the understanding of written language.

In some cases, the patient's reading performance can also be improved by altering the conditions of presentation. For instance, Beringer and Stein's patient (1930) could read many more words if they were presented one at a time, on a bright screen in a dark room, and if, in addition, she was allowed to rest after each stimulus. Enhancing visual stimulation and avoiding fatigue then may result in better reading.

2.1.10. *Silent versus Oral Reading*

More often than not pure alexics perform better on silent reading than on oral reading tasks. For instance, the patient of Stachowiak and Poeck (1976) could not read aloud a single word, but he was correct 72.5% of the time when in a series of 4 written words he had to choose the one that corresponded to an object he was palpating, and 77% when he had to choose the word that had been mentioned orally by the examiner. The patient described by Lebrun and Devreux (1983) could generally match written words with pictures, although she could not always read these words aloud correctly. For instance, she appropriately matched the word "cigarettes" with a picture representing a box of cigarettes, but she said: "Fish, fishing."

Correct identification with false naming was also observed in Caplan and Hedley-Whyte's case (1974). For instance, the patient managed to order some ten letters in alphabetical order but misnamed most of them. She would generally complete letters adequately in words or appropriately cover extra letters with her hand, although she read the words aloud erroneously. For instance, being shown the anomalous word "CATAT", she covered the last two letters, but said: "Boy."

A similar discrepancy between silent and oral reading was also noted in the case reported by Albert *et al.* (1973). The patient was shown a single written word and was asked to select from among three pictures the one that corrersponded to the word. He selected the correct alternative in eight of ten items of this kind. However, he could read aloud correctly only three of the eight words he had appropriately matched with the picture. One of his failures concerned the word "shoe"; he pointed to the correct picture but said: "I can't name it. I can't name it. I can't read it. I know what it is. I can't read." He then tried to identify the individual letters which the word comprised, but he erred completely: "g-m-o-a, t-o-m-o". On another occasion, he was shown a picture of a lion and was requested to point to the correct word from among the written alternatives "cat", "lion", and "bear". He correctly designated the word "lion", but read it aloud as "Black. No. Horse, I imagine. Yeah, black".

The patient of Dünsing (1953a) had occasional difficulty in reading letters aloud. The letter "L" she found every time difficult to identify by name. She recognized it, as she could tell that it was her problem letter and also the initial of her husband's first name (Ludwig). Still, she had great difficulty in naming it.

Actually, the reading aloud of letters and of words is a naming on confrontation task (Figure 2), different from the silent identification of written material. In pure alexia, the former is usually more disturbed than the latter. Accordingly, pure alexics generally make less errors when pointing to letters or words mentioned by the examiner than when reading letters or words aloud.

2.1.11. *Perseveration*

In reading aloud, alexic patients may give perseverative responses. It is not always clear whether these perseverations are efferent or afferent in nature, that is, whether the patient has recognized that the second stimulus is different from the first one but cannot help giving it the same name (output problem) or whether he thinks that he has been presented the

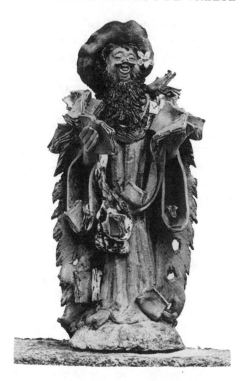

Fig. 2. Reading aloud.

same stimulus two times in succession (input problem). For instance, Alajouanine (1968, p. 128) mentions a French-speaking patient who was once requested to read aloud the following passage (the first sentence was the title of the passage): "Pierre se casse une jambe. Après le jour de l'an, il fit très froid. Les enfants ne sortirent plus. La mare de la ferme gela." The patient said: "Pierre se lasse dans la lance. Après le jour de l'an, la fin que les enfants ne sont plus la lance de sa lance lance sur la sur de la terre, de la terre sur. . . ." Alajouanine also mentions a patient who had the impression, when his alexia set in, that all the articles in his newspaper began with the same sentence.

2.1.12. *Visual Problems*

Alexics may not only have perceptual perseverations when looking at written material, they may also find it difficult to focus on print or script. They may complain that the written words they are looking at are not stable, seems to "spill down" or to "fall of the side of the page". The patient of Ajax (1967) reported "shuddering" of individual words as he attempted to decipher them. Patients may also have difficulty in making the transition from one line of print to another.

2.1.13. *Figures and Numbers*

Not infrequently, the reading of figures and even of numbers is better preserved than that of letters and words. For instance, Hinshelwood (1902) mentioned a patient who despite global alexia could "read figures up to millions with correctness and fluency" and the patient of Ajax (1967) despite his verbal alexia could deal with figures and mathematical formulas. However, in some instances digits cause as much trouble as letters. For instance, the first patient of Boudouresques *et al.*, (1972) made nearly as many errors in reading figures and numbers as in reading letters and words. And the first patient of Lebrun *et al.*, (1979), because he could no longer handle figures, was unable to dial telephone numbers.

Telling the time may also be affected, as in the first case reported by Lebrun *et al.* (1979). Interestingly, reading a clock may be impossible or incorrect, even though the patient can identify individual digits, as the case of Fincham *et al.* (1975) shows. This patient was also unable to use calendars. On the other hand, the ability to tell the time may be totally preserved even in the presence of global alexia, as the case of Baruk *et al.* (1928) shows.

2.1.14. *Other Visual Codes*

The interpretation of visual codes other than written language may or may not be disturbed. For instance, the first of the four alexics described by Hinshelwood (1902) could read musical notes without any difficulty. On the contrary, Dejerine's patient (1892) had completely lost the ability to read scores. The second patient of Lebrun *et al.* (1979) and the patient of Pillon *et al.* (1987) could no longer interpret highway signs correctly whereas the patient of Warrington and Zangwill (1957) could still do so. The patient of Fincham *et al.* (1975) could correctly name the colours of traffic lights but confused their meanings. As for the patient of Michel *et al.* (1979), he could no longer use playing cards.

2.1.15. *Identifying Words Spelled Aloud by the Examiner*

A number of pure alexics (e.g., the patients of Bramwell, 1897, of Boudouresques *et al.*, 1972, and of Greenblatt, 1976) can recognize words that are verbally spelled for them. Others (e.g., the first patient of Lebrun *et al.*, 1979) find this task difficult. Clinical reality then is complex and partly falsifies Benson and Geschwind's statement (1969) that "the

114   YVAN LEBRUN AND LUC DE VREESE

patient with alexia without agraphia readily comprehends words spelled aloud to him by the examiner".

2.2. *Writing*

In patients with pure alexia, there typically is a striking contrast between reading and writing. This does not mean that writing is totally normal. Generally, it is not, but errors in writing are far less numerous than in reading. Moreover, the patient appears to write fluently, without undue effort, whereas reading, if at all possible, is laborious.

Writing errors made by pure alexics may be misspellings. These orthographic errors may be due, at least in part, to the patient's inability to read over what he has been writing and thus to correct his mistakes.

In addition to spelling errors, pure alexics not infrequently make duplications or omissions of letters and/or of strokes. For instance, the samples reproduced by Dejerine (1892) show that the patient doubled the "i" in the French word for cold, "froid" and wrote an "m" with four downstrokes in the French word "novembre". The first patient of Dejerine and Pelissier (1914) wrote an "m" with only two downstrokes in the French word "empresse" and omitted the "r" at the end of "monsieur".

Besides these duplications and deletions, there may be abnormal spacing of letters within words, the lines of script may not be horizontal (as in Dünsing's case, 1953a), or letters may be written over one another (as in Dejerine's case, 1892). These features are somewhat reminiscent of afferent agraphia as it is frequently observed in nonalexic patients with right brain damage (Lebrun, 1985) and may be due, in cases of pure alexia, to the absence of adequate visual control in writing. As a matter of fact, Dejerine's patient (1892) complained that he could not check what he was writing. Indeed, trying to read what he was penning made him confused and prevented him from proceeding with writing.

Attentive reading of published cases of pure alexia strongly suggests that very few patients can be said to have had intact writing skills. Complete preservation of writing abilities in the presence of pure alexia seems extremely rare indeed. Accordingly, when one refers to pure alexia as "alexia without agraphia", one should be aware of the fact that this phrase in fact means "alexia without commensurate agraphia".

When the alexia is global or primarily literal, forming words with anagram letters is difficult, as the letters have to be identified before they can be selected and properly ordered. When given the letters he needed the patient of Gloning *et al.* (1955) ordered them correctly but put some of them upside down or sideways. In the first case reported by Dejerine and Pélissier (1914), the identification of letters was slow but usually correct. Accordingly, the patient could form words with anagram letters if given enough time.

Pure alexics are typically unable to read over what they have written once the memory of it has ceased to operate. They may be able to distinguish their own handwriting from someone else's, though. However, this is not always the case, as the paper by Hirose *et al.* (1977) shows.

2.2.1. *Copying*

Whereas writing spontaneously or to dictation is fluent, copying is generally arduous in pure alexia. The patients work slowly, painfully endeavouring to reproduce the model. Their performance is usually poor. For instance, the patient of Dejerine (1892) could not even copy single block letters correctly. And the handwriting of the patient described by Gallois *et al.* (1988) became illegible when she was made to copy written words. Some patients seem unable to reproduce printed letters faithfully, as they attempt to replace them by cursive letters, as in Dejerine and Pélissier's first case (1914).

In a few cases, the dyscopia was found to be unilateral. For instance, a right-handed Japanese observed by Yamadori (1980) could copy Japanese characters (kana and kanji) correctly with the left but not with the right hand. Caplan and Hedley-Whyte's right-handed patient (1974) too could copy correctly with her left hand. Right-sided paresis prevented testing of the right hand.

However, there are pure alexics who can copy normally with their preferred hand, as the case reported by Crouzon and Valence shows (1923).

2.2.2. *Transcribing*

Turning script into print or vice-versa may or may not be possible. For instance, in the case reported by Pillon *et al.* (1987) the patient quickly recovered the ability to perform such a task despite the persistence of alexia.

2.2.3. *Spelling Aloud Words Specified by the Examiner*

Pure alexics may or may not be able to spell aloud correctly words specified by the examiner. The patients of Boudouresques *et al.* (1972) and the patient of Gallois *et al.* (1988) made no mistake while spelling aloud from memory, although their alexia was severe. By contrast, the first patient of Lebrun *et al.* (1979) made mistakes when spelling aloud words, although premorbidly he had had a good command of orthography. Clinical reality then does not fully bear out Benson and Geschwind's statement (1969) that "the patient with alexia without agraphia spells aloud correctly".

2.2.4. *Detecting Spelling Errors*

The patient of Pillon *et al.* (1987) whose alexia was primarily verbal could detect spelling errors in written words when he was told what the words were.

2.3. *Color Aphasia*

Many patients with pure alexia make errors when naming colors on confrontation. To a lesser extent, they also have trouble to point to colors mentioned by the examiner. A few of them make mistakes when they have to indicate verbally the typical color of objects specified by the examiner (such as snow, blood, coal, etc.). All these patients have color aphasia in addition to their alexia. In some cases, the color aphasia results from a visuo-verbal dissociation: color names can no longer be properly associated with visual percepts. In other cases, the color aphasia is a category-specific aphasia: the use of color names is selectively disturbed.

Patients with color aphasia not infrequently give bizarre answers when asked to name plain colors. For instance, when shown a plainly yellow pencil and asked what the color of it was, Greenblatt's patient (1976) hesitated for many seconds and then said: "sort of orangish-yellow".

Patients with color aphasia may have some degree of color agnosia. In such a case, they make mistakes when coloring outline drawings of objects having a typical color (such as a lemon) or when in an array of differently colored representations of a familiar object, they have to select the representation with the appropriate color. The first patient of Boudouresques *et al.* (1972) and the patient of Lhermitte and Beauvois (1973) had some degree of color agnosia in addition to their color aphasia.

2.4. *Optic or Visual Aphasia*

In a number of cases (e.g., the second patient of Boudourseques *et al.* 1972, and the patient of Lebrun and Devreux, 1984) the difficulty to name on confrontation extends to objects and to pictures of objects. These patients have optic or visual aphasia. This is a modality-specific aphasia. The patient with optic aphasia makes mistakes when naming objects presented visually while he names them correctly if he is allowed to palpate or to hear them. He can correctly mime the use of the objects which he cannot name. He can also give the names of objects which are verbally described by the examiner.

Wernicke in 1886 was already aware of the possibility of there being visual aphasia in cases of pure alexia. Sometimes, as in the first case reported by Boudouresques *et al.* (1972), there is optic aphasia for pictures but not for three-dimensional objects.

Generally, patients with optic aphasia perform better on the pointing than on the naming test.

Patients with optic aphasia may, as in the case reported by Lebrun and Devreux (1984), also have some degree of visual agnosia; that is to say, in addition to their difficulty in naming objects presented visually, they at times fail to recognize objects shown or mistake them for others. In such cases, only careful examination can discover the errors due to optic aphasia and those due to visual agnosia.

2.5. *Other Neurolinguistic Deficits*

In adddition to, or apart from, color aphasia and optic aphasia, there may be slight aphasic deficits affecting comprehension of complex orders or list generation. There may also be slight to moderate word-finding difficulties, especially as regards proper names (e.g., Dünsing, 1953a; Lebrun *et al.*, 1979, first case). The patient of Gallois *et al.* (1988) could never remember the names of celebrities though she could identify them. A slight anomia was also observed by Boudouresques *et al.* (1972) in their first case.

There may also be a reduction of short-term verbal memory. In some cases, the reduction is marked.

In fact, no case of pure alexia seems to have ever been described in which the linguistic impairment was strictly limited to reading skills. In all reported patients, other verbal functions were affected at the same time, though to a much lesser extent. The appellation "pure alexia" therefore should be taken to mean: "relatively pure alexia". It refers to a condition in which the reading disorder is disproportionate to, or far more incapacitating than, the other neurolinguistic deficits.

2.6. *Hemifield Alexia*

A few patients have been reported who made more errors when having to name letters, words and digits flashed to one of their visual hemifields than when the same stimuli were flashed to the other hemifield. Such patients are sometimes said to have "hemifield alexia" (e.g., Castro-Caldas and Salgado, 1984). This specific kind of pure alexia has been observed in a number of subjects having undergone surgical transsection of their corpus callosum (Greenblatt, 1977).

2.7. *Nonverbal Deficits*

A number of nonlinguistic deficits may accompany pure alexia. For instance, there may be dyscalculia (as in the first case reported by Lebrun *et al.*, 1979). The calculation disorder may occur even if the patient can read numbers correctly, as Hinshelwood's first case shows.

On the other hand, some patients can still calculate mentally even though they are alexic for figures and numbers (as in the case reported by Crouzon and Valence, 1923).

Drawing may be disturbed. Indeed, there may be constructional apraxia.

Pure alexics may also show some degree of simultanagnosia, as in the case described by Gloning *et al.* (1955). Patients with simultagnosia can see the details of a complex scene but fail to recognize the scene as a whole.

There may also be topographical disorientation as well as left-right confusion.

Last but not least, memory disturbances, expecially for recent events, have been noted in a number of pure alexics. There may also be reduced ability to remember digits presented by the examiner.

As a matter of fact, careful investigation of pure alexics nearly always brings a number of nonverbal cognitive deficits to light. From a neuropsychological point of view pure alexics are rarely, if ever, monosymptomatic. This remark holds good in respect of neurology. The neurological examination of pure alexics is seldom or never entirely normal. Probably the most frequently encountered deficit relates to vision.

2.8. *Visual Defects*

As early as 1886 Wernicke posited that right-sided hemianopia was a regular (he said "gesetzmässig") accompaniment of pure alexia. This view was echoed by Dejerine and Pélissier in 1914. However, a number of cases have been reported which had pure alexia without hemianopia or even quadranopia (e.g., Hinshelwood, 1902, case No. 1; Greenblatt, 1973; Vincent *et al.*, 1977). In the case described by Ajax (1967) the hemianopia, which was present at onset, cleared after some time, while the alexia remained.

When hemianopia is present, it is generally on the right side, but a few cases have been reported who had left hemianopia (e.g., Gloning *et al.*, 1955; Fincham *et al.*, 1975; Pillon *et al.*, 1987). The hemianopia is usally homonymous — that is to say, the two right, or two left, visual hemifields are similarly affected.

Occasionally the hemianopia is not absolute in that stimuli presented in the affected hemifields are perceived but only dimly. For instance, Dejerine's patient (1892) could faintly see objects presented in his right hemifields but they appeared colorless. This man then had right-sided hemiachromatopsia — that is to say that he was unable to perceive colors in his right hemifields.

The right-sided hemianopia may result in the patient failing to see the rightmost letters of the words. However, this cannot account for most of the reading difficulties of pure alexics. For instance, the patient of Dünsing (1953b) could read numbers which his visual field defect prevented him from seeing in their totality in one fixation, but he had much difficulty in reading short monosyllables which he could see wholly in one fixation.

In addition to hemianopia there may be an oculor motor disturbance, as in the case described by Warrington and Zangwill (1957).

2.9. *Other Neurological Accompaniments*

Sensory deficits in the form of hemihypoesthesia have been observed in a number of patients. Occasionally, there was also a unilateral motor disorder, as in Caplan and Hedley-Whyte's case (1974).

3. CLINICO-ANATOMICAL CORRELATIONS

In the majority of the reported cases of pure alexia, the cause appeared to be a vascular accident in the territory of the posterior cerebral artery. Most of the time the medial and inferior aspects of the occipital lobe and the splenium — i.e., the posterior part of the corpus callosum — were infracted. In a few cases, however, the splenium was spared (e.g., Hécaen and Gruner, 1974).

Several cases have also been reported in which pure alexia resulted from a cerebral trauma (e.g., Baruk *et al.*, 1928; Franceschetti and de Morsier, 1937) or a tumour (e.g., Greenblatt, 1973; Vincent *et al.*, 1977) or appeared after an arteriovenous malformation had been surgically removed (Ajax, 1967).

In all cases, the lesion involved the posterior part of at least one hemisphere. When cerebral damage was unilateral, it was most of the time on the left. Only few cases of unilateral right brain damage have been reported. For instance, Pillon *et al.*, (1987) observed pure alexia in a left-hander after a stroke in the territory of the right posterior cerebral artery. By contrast, the patient of Hirose *et al.* (1977), who had pure alexia secondary to a right vascular occipital lesion, was right-handed. This man then had crossed pure alexia.

4. PATHOGENESIS

As early as 1886 Carl Wernicke posited that pure alexia, which he called "subcortical alexia", was due to an interruption of the pathways leading from the end station of the optic tract to the center containing the images of written words.

In 1892 Jules Dejerine reported a case of pure alexia which he had been able to autopsy. There was a lesion in the medial and inferior aspects of the left occipital lobe and another in the posterior part of the corpus callosum. Dejerine considered that the occipital lesion was responsible for the alexia as it interrupted the optic radiations to the left visual cortex, the fibers connecting the right visual cortex with the left visual cortex, and the fibers connecting the left visual cortex with the angular gyrus (Figure 3).

In 1925 Foix and Hillemand reported the case of a man in whom a cerebrovascular accident had deeply infarcted the left occipital lobe but had completely spared the corpus callosum. This lesion had not resulted in alexia. Foix and Hillemand concluded that a lesion of the splenium, i.e., the posterior part of the corpus callosum, was necessary for there to be pure alexia.

While he greatly valued Dejerine's neuropathological report of 1892, Geschwind (1962, 1965) shared the view of Foix and Hillemand that the

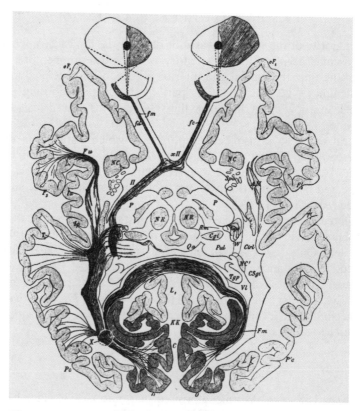

Fig. 3. "X" denotes the intra-hemispheric lesion which Dejerine (1892) considered to be responsible for pure alexia.

splenial lesion was as important as the left occipital lesion in the pathogenesis of pure alexia.

In fact, Geschwind and the neo-associationist school have construed
pure alexia as a prototypic instance of disconnection. The disconnection
theory of alexia without agraphia implies that visual information about
written material reaching the calcarine areas cannot be relayed to the
dominant angular gyrus to be decoded, either because this gyrus has been
undercut by the lesion or because a double lesion has destroyed both the
ipsilateral visual cortex and the splenium or its outflow. When the lesion
undercuts the angular gyrus, some speak of "subangular alexia" which they
contrast with "splenioccipital alexia".

The disconnection theory of pure alexia has been widely accepted. Yet,
it fails to account well for a number of clinical observations. For instance,
how can it explain that a number of pure alexics have not the slightest
difficulty in naming objects perceived visually? If, as the theory implies,
the brain damage which these patients have incurred prevents their
dominant hemisphere from seeing objects (hemianopia) and if visual
information cannot be relayed from the non-dominant visual cortex to the
language zone in the dominant hemisphere because of the splenial lesion,
how do the patients manage to name objects perceived by their non-
dominant visual cortex? Geschwind (1965) attempted to answer this
question by pointing out that most objects can not only be seen but also
handled. It may therefore be conjectured that the visual perception of a
familiar object immediately arouses tactile associations in the brain.
Specifically, when the nondominant visual cortex perceives an object, this
percept arouses tactile associations in the parietal cortex on the same side.
The excited parietal neurons may then communicate with the language
zone on the other side of the brain, using undamaged anterior callosal
fibers.

If this explanation is valid, then it may be presumed that tactile
sensations reaching the parietal cortex when an object is held by the left
hand, arouse visual associations in the ipsilateral visual cortex. Accordingly, if an anterior callosal lesion prevents tactile information from
travelling directly from the non-dominant parietal cortex to the language
zone on the dominant side, the detour via the ipsilateral visual cortex and
the splenium should be possible. Unfortunately, clinical findings fail to
bear out this hypothesis. For instance, Geschwind and Kaplan (1962)
reported the case of a right-handed man with left tactile aphasia. This
patient constantly misnamed objects palpated with his left hand, although
his pantomime clearly indicated that he had duly recognized these objects.
Geschwind and Kaplan assumed that the cause of the disorder was
damage to the anterior part of the corpus callosum. If this assumption is
correct, why could this man in tactile naming not use the route from the

right parietal cortex (the end station of the tactile pathways from the left hand) to the right visual cortex and from there to the left language zone via the splenium, which in his case, seemed intact? It follows from all this that the disconnection theory does not satisfactorily explain the occurrence of pure alexia without visual aphasia.

The theory also fails to account for the fact that a number of pure alexics have no difficulty in naming colors or in reading aloud numbers. Colors and numbers can hardly be said to have tactile associations. How is it then that they can be named while letters and/or words cannot? The problem can be solved by assuming that the splenial fibers form groups, each of which is specialized in the transmission of a specific kind of material: one bundle for written language, another for colors, and yet another for figures. However, the identification of these bundles proves difficult. For instance, Ajax *et al.* (1977) ascribed the absence of color aphasia in their alexic patient to the intactness of the superior part of the splenium, whereas Vincent *et al.* (1977) ascribed it, in their case, to the intactness of the dorsal part of the splenium.

Another problem with the concept of specialized transcollosal visual fibers is that it does not explain why the bundle for figures and numbers tends to be less frequently or less severely damaged than the bundle for letters and words.

Last but not least, the assumed specialization does not account for the fact that Hinshelwood's first patient (1902) was nearly totally alexic for English, partially alexic for French and Latin, and virtually not alexic for Greek. One can hardly presume that he had transcallosal fibers which were used for the transmission of written Greek, others for the transmission of written Latin or French, and still others for the transmission of written English.

Dyscopia is yet another thorny problem. To be sure, its presence can be explained in terms of disconnection. One may reason that if the patient has right homonymous hemianopia, he can only perceive the model to be reproduced with his right visual cortex. Therefore, if he is right-handed, instructions for copying have to travel from the right visual cortex to the left motor strip via the corpus callosum. If the latter is damaged, the transmission of these instruction, i.e., the visuo-motor coordination, is impaired and dyscopia obtains.

Such a view accords well with the fact that the alexic patients of Yamadori (1980) and of Assal and Regli (1980) were dyscopic with their right hand but not with their left; copying with the left hand did not involve any transcallosal transfer and could therefore be adequately performed.

The theory also explains why some pure alexics attempt to read what they are to copy instead of simply reproducing it; they try to decode the words so that their left hemisphere can know what is to be reproduced and can guide their right hand as it does when the patients write spontaneously or to dictation.

However, the theory does not account well for the fact that some pure alexics with right hemianopia have no difficulty in copying with their right hand, as in Crouzon and Valence's case (1923). How is it that in these patients the visuo-motor coordination is not disturbed? How are the visual information transmitted from the right visual cortex to the left motor strip? The disconnection theory provides no answer. Unless, of course, one assumes that in cases of pure alexia with right hemianopia but no dyscopia, the right hand is directed by the right hemisphere using un-crossed pyramidal tracts. So far, however, no evidence has been adduced in support of this hypothesis.

The case reported by Fincham *et al.* (1975) is also difficult to reconcile with the disconnection theory. Their patient was a right-handed scholar who, at autopsy, was found to have several metastatic lesions, none of which damaged the left occipital lobe or undercut the left angular gyrus. On the right, the splenium and large portions of the right hemisphere were involved. Such a case is difficult to interpret in the light of the disconnec-tion model, unless one assumes that in that right-handed patient, the right hemisphere was dominant for language. However, this hypothesis does not fit in well with the fact that despite massive destruction of the posterior part of his right, supposedly dominant, hemisphere, this man had no aphasia.

The disconnection theory then accounts for some clinical observations and leaves others unexplained. Probably the pathophysiology of pure alexia is too complex to be completely accountable in terms of disruption of pathways. Geschwind (1974) himself seems to have realized this, as he stated at a meeting in Lyon, France, that the concept of disconnection was useful in the study of brain pathology but could not be expected to uncover intricate brain mechanisms.

5. PROGNOSIS AND THERAPY

The evolution of pure alexia resembles its symptomatology in that it shows important interindividual differences. In a number of cases, spontaneous recovery is observed. For instance, the alexia of Dejerine and Pélissier's second patient (1914), which was severe initially, cleared after a few months.

In other cases, significant improvement can be achieved through therapy. For instance, a four stage therapy designed by Beauvois and Dérouesné (1982) helped a 61-year-old patient regain enough reading skills to understand novels.

Other patients, on the contrary, fail to recover usable reading skills even after prolonged training. For instance, in the case reported by Ajax (1967), "despite extraordinary efforts on the part of the patient and devoted assistance by others, no significant improvement occurred". Notwithstand-ing sustained efforts Dejerine's patient (1892) also failed to recover the ability to read text or scores. In such cases, it is not clear whether the alexia was totally incurable or whether a different therapeutic approach could have proved more fruitful. In Beauvois and Dérouesné's case, improvement did not begin until a new therapy tailored to the patient's specific difficulties had been substituted for a more traditional approach.

6. CONCLUSIONS AND SUMMARY

Damage to the posterior part of the brain may result in a rather severe reading impairment. This disorder is usally accompanied by other, less conspicuous, neurolinguistic or cognitive deficits.

In some cases, letters and words are equally difficult to identify or to sound out. In other cases, the reading of letters and the reading of words are differently affected. The reading of figures and of numbers is often less impaired than that of letters and words. The decoding of other visual codes may or may not be disordered. Thus, the symptomatology of pure alexia is far from being uniform.

The etiopathology of the condition has not yet been completely eluci-dated. The disconnection model, which is often used to explain the disorder, does not account for all the observed facts. Indeed, due to interindividual differences in cerebral organization and disorganization, it is unlikely that a unitary theory can ever be developed that can satis-factorily account for all the various features of pure alexia.

Diversity is also present in the rate of recovery. The disorder may clear spontaneously, regress under the influence of treatment, or prove therapy-resistant.

Pure alexia then beautifully epitomizes the complexity and intricacy of disturbances of higher cerebral functions.

REFERENCES

Ajax, E.: 1967, 'Dyslexia without agraphia', *Archives of Neurology* **17**, 645—652.
Ajax, E., Schenkenberg, T. and Kosteljanetz, M.: 1977, 'Alexia without agraphia and the inferior planum', *Neurology* **27**, 685—688.
Alajouanine, T.: 1968, *L'aphasie et le Langage Pathologique*, Baillière, Paris.
Albert, M., Yamadori, A., Gardner, H. and Howes, D.: 1973, 'Comprehension in alexia', *Brain* **96**, 317—328.
Assal, G. and Regli, F.: 1980, 'Syndrome de disconnexion visuo-verbale et visuo-gestuelle. Aphasie optique et apraxie optique', *Revue Neurologique* **136**, 365—376.
Assal, G. and Zander, E.: 1975, 'Anomie et alexie lors d'un traumatisme cranio-cérébral fermé', *Neuro-Chirurgie* **21**, 591—596.
Baruk, H., Bertrand, I. and Hartmann, E.: 1928, 'Un cas d'alexie traumatique', *Revue Neurologique* , 287—292.
Beauvois, M. F. and Dérouesné, J.: 1982, 'Recherche en neuropsychologie et rééducation. Quels rapports?', in Seron, X. and Laterre, C. (eds.), *Rééduquer le Cerveau*, Mardaga, Brussels, pp. 163—189.

Benson, F. and Geschwind, N.: 1969, 'The alexias', in Vinken, P. and Bruyn, G. (eds.), *Handbook of Clinical Neurology*, Vol. 4, pp. 112—140. North Holland Publishing Company, Amsterdam.

Beringer, K. and Stein, J.: 1930, 'Analyse eines Falles von "reiner" Alexie', *Zeitschrift für Neurologie* **123**, 472—478.

Botez, M. and Serbanescu, T.: 1967, 'Course and outcome of visual static agnosia', *Journal of the Neurological Sciences* **4**, 289—297.

Botez, M., Serbanescu, T. and Vernea, I.: 1964, 'Visual static agnosia with special reference to literal agnosic alexia', *Neurology* **14**, 1101—1111.

Boudouresques, J., Poncet, M., Sebahoun, M. and Alicherif, A.: 1972, 'Deux cas d'alexie sans agraphie avec troubles de la dénomination des couleurs et des images', *Oto-Neuro-Ophtalmologie* **44**, 297—304.

Bramwell, B.: 1897, 'Illustrative cases of aphasia', *Lancet* **75** (March 27), 868—871.

Caplan, L. and Hedley-Whyte, T.: 1974, 'Cuing and memory dysfunction in alexia without agraphia', *Brain* **97**, 251—262.

Castro-Caldas, A. and Salgado, V.: 1984, 'Right hemifield alexia without hemianopia', *Archives of Neurology* **41**, 84—87.

Crouzon, X. and Valence, X.: 1923, 'Un cas d'alexie pure', *Semaine des Hôpitaux de Paris* **47**, 1145—1149.

Cumming, W., Hurwitz, L. and Perl, N.: 1970, 'A study of a patient who had alexia without agraphia', *Journal of Neurology, Neurosurgery, and Psychiatry* **33**, 34—39.

Dejerine, J.: 1892, 'Contribution à l'étude anatomo-pathologique et clinique des différentes variétés de cécité verbale', *Mémoires de la Société de Biologie* **4**, 61—90.

Dejerine, J. and Pélissier, A.: 1914, 'Contribution à l'étude de la cécité verbale pure', *L'Encéphale* **9** (7), 1—28.

Dide, M. and Botcazo, X.: 1902, 'Amnésie continue, cécité verbale pure, perte du sens topographique, ramollissement double du lobe lingual', *Revue Neurologique* **00**, 676—680.

Dünsing, F.: 1953a, 'Zur Frage der Buchstabenalexie', *Zeitschrift für Psychiatrie* **191**, 147—162.

Dünsing, F.: 1953b, 'Ueber die Wortalexie', *Archiv für Psychiatrie* **191**, 163—178.

Fincham, R., Nibbelinck, D. and Aschenbrenner, C.: 1975, 'Alexia with left homonymous hemianopia without agraphia', *Neurology* **25**, 1164—1168.

Foix, C. and Hillemand, P.: 1925, 'Rôle vraisemblable du splénium dans la pathogénie de l'alexie pure par lésion de la cérébrale postérieure', *Semaine des Hôpitaux de Paris* **49**, 393—395.

Franceschetti, A. and de Morsier, G.: 1937, 'Un cas d'alexie pure d'origine traumatique avec hémianopsie en cadran inférieur droit', *Revue d'Oto-Neuro-Ophtalmologie* **16**, 125—127.

Gallois, P., Ovelacq, E., Hautecœvr, P. and Dereux, J.: 1988, 'Disconnexion et reconnaissance des visages', *Revue Neurologique* **144**, 113—119.

Geschwind, N.: 1962, 'The anatomy of acquired disorders of reading', in Money, J. (ed.), *Reading Disability*, pp. 115—129, The Johns Hopkins Press, Baltimore.

Geschwind, N.: 1965, 'Disconnexion syndromes in animals and man', *Brain* **88**, 237—294, 585—644.

Geschwind, N.: 1974, 'Le concept de disconnexion: L'histoire d'une idée banale mais importante', in Michel, F. and Schott, B. (eds.), *Les Syndromes de Disconnexion Calleuse chez l'Homme*, pp. 11—15, Lyon.

Geschwind, N. and Kaplan, E.: 1962, 'A human cerebral deconnection syndrome', *Neurology* **12**, 675—685.

Gloning, I., Gloning, K., Seitelberger, F. and Tschabitscher, H.: 1955, 'Ein Fall von reiner Wortblindheit mit Obduktionsbefund', *Wiener Zeitschrift für Nervenheilkunde* **12**, 194—215.

Greenblatt, S.: 1973, 'Alexia without agraphia or hemianopia: Anatomical analysis of an autopsied case', *Brain* **96**, 307—316.
Greenblatt, S.: 1976, 'Subangular alexia without agraphia or hemianopsia', *Brain and Language* **3**, 229—245.
Greenblatt, S.: 1977, 'Neurosurgery and the anatomy of reading: A practical review', *Neurosurgery* **1**, 6—15.
Hécaen, H. and Gruner, J.: 1974, 'Alexie "pure" avec intégrité du corps calleux', in Michel, F. and Schott, B. (eds.), *Les Syndromes de Disconnexion Calleuse chez l'Homme*, pp. 347—361, Lyon.
Hinshelwood, J.: 1902, 'Four cases of word-blindness', *Lancet* **1**, 358—363.
Hirose, G., Kin, T. and Murakami, E.: 1977, 'Alexia without agraphia associated with right occipital lesion', *Journal of Neurology, Neurosurgery and Psychiatry* **40**, 225—227.
Lebrun, Y.: 1985, 'Disturbances of written language and associated abilities following damage to the right hemisphere', *Applied Psycholinguistics* **6**, 231—260.
Lebrun, Y. and Devreux, F.: 1984, 'Alexia in relation to aphasia and agnosia', in Malatesha, R. and Whitaker, H. (eds.), *Dyslexia: A Global Issue*, pp. 191—209, Nijhoff, The Hague.
Lebrun, Y., Hoops, R., Monseu, G., Collier, A. and Stoupel, N.: 1979, 'Pure word blindness: An overview', in Lebrun, Y. and Hoops, R. (eds.), *Problems of Aphasia*, pp. 79—93, Swets and Zeitlinger, Lisse.
Lhermitte, F. and Beauvois M.: 1973, 'A visual-speech disconnexion syndrome', *Brain* **96**, 695—714.
Marie, P.: 1906a, 'La troisième circonvolution frontale gauche ne joue aucun rôle spécial dans la fonction du langage', *La Semaine Médicale* **26**, 241—247.
Marie, P.: 1906b, 'Que faut-il penser des aphasies sous-corticales?', *La Semaine Médicale* **26**, 493—500.
Michel, F., Schott, B., Boucher, M. and Kopp, N.: 1979, 'Alexie sans agraphie chez un malade ayant un hémisphère gauche déafférenté', *Revue Neurologique* **135**, 347—364.
Ombredane, A.: 1944, *Etude de Psychologie Médicale*, Atlantica Editora, Rio de Janeiro.
Pillon, B., Bakchine, S. and Lhermitte, F.: 1987, 'Alexia without agraphia in a left-handed patient with a right occipital lesion', *Archives of Neurology* **44**, 1257—1262.
Sasanuma, S.: 1974, 'Kanji versus kana processing in alexia with transient agraphia: A case report', *Cortex* **10**, 89—97.
Stachowiak, F. and Poeck, K.: 1976, 'Functional disconnection in pure alexia and color naming deficit demonstrated by facilitating methods', *Brain and Language* **3**, 135—143.
Vincent, F., Sadowsky, C., Saunders, R. and Reeves, A.: 1977, 'Alexia without agraphia, hemianopia, or color-naming defect: A disconnection syndrome', *Neurology* **27**, 689—691.
Warrington, E. and Zangwill, O.: 1957, 'A study of dyslexia', *Journal of Neurology, Neurosurgery and Psychiatry* **20**, 208—215.
Wernicke, C.: 1886, 'Die neueren Arbeiten über Aphasie', *Fortschritte der Medizin* **4**, 371—377, 463—482.
Yamadori, A.: 1980, 'Right unilateral dyscopia of letters in alexia without agraphia', *Neurology* **30**, 991—994.

WRITER'S CRAMP

1. INTRODUCTION

In September 1872, a British medical journal called *The Practitioner* published a paper by George Vivian Poore which contained the description of a right-handed bachelor named George Gair, who had been a clerk first in a commercial firm and then in an accountant's office. There, by reason of his neat handwriting, he had been constantly employed in copying balance sheets. He used to do, on average, nine hours of writing a day. He had been working in this way for about 14 months when one evening, towards the close of his day's work, he experienced some difficulty in keeping his right hand on the sheet. This difficulty remained all through the following three days. In order to write he had to hold his right hand firmly on the desk with his left hand.

During the subsequent month the writing impediment increased until George found himself totally unable to write with his right hand. He could perform all other unimanual activities as before.

Because he could no longer make his preferred hand hold the pen and form letters, he taught himself to write with his left hand and for 10 years used that hand to do his writing. Then his left hand too lost the ability to form letters. At the same time, his right hand started to have spasms during the performance of such actions as cutting meat with a knife or pouring water out of a jug. After some time, the hand became subject to constant twitching whether it was active or at rest. It was at that time that he was examined by Poore, who asked him to write his name with his preferred hand.

He takes the pen in hand [Poore reported] and immediately he does so there is a violent cramp of the triceps, the arm is forcibly extended, and with great difficulty he manages to write "Geor" in a manner scarcely legible, when the hand is twisted off the paper by a violent rotation of the wrist and his fingers lose the grasp of the pen. On asking him to continue writing, he is perfectly unable to do so, and every effort even to place his hand on the paper seems to be violently resisted by every muscle from the deltoid downwards.

This report is one of the first detailed descriptions that can be found of a writing impediment ordinarily called *writer's cramp* or *writers' cramp*. Other, less common names, are *scrivener's palsy, graphospasm,* and *mogigraphia.*

Since the publication of Poore's paper in 1872, the various features of writer's cramp have been analyzed and it is possible at present to give a

R. M. Joshi (ed.), Written Language Disorders, 127—142.
© 1991 *Kluwer Academic Publishers. Printed in the Netherlands.*

survey of the different forms which this curious disorder of graphomotricity may take.

2. SYMPTOMATOLOGY

2.1. *Writing Impairment*

In patients with writer's cramp writing is rendered difficult by a tonic spasm, dystonia, dyskinesia, tremor, akinesia, loss of motor control, or by a combination of these. In cases with tonic spasm, the hand and fingers, and sometimes also the wrist, stiffen. This muscular contraction may or may not be painful. If present, the pain may involve the hand and fingers only or, on the contrary, spread to the whole upper limb including the shoulder. Occasionally, as in the case reported by Martinez-Martin and Pareja (1984), stiffness and pain are felt in the forearm and wrist, to the exclusion of the hand. On the whole, the pain tends to spread more than the spasm itself. In addition to the cramp, there may be abnormal palmar sweating.

Sometimes the involuntary contraction causes the hand or forearm to assume a position inappropriate for writing. For instance, in a case reported by Ravits *et al.* (1985), involuntary supination of the forearm came about whenever the patient engaged in writing.

In addition to dystonia (= abnormal state of contraction and abnormal posture), there may be involuntary jerks of the fingers or hand. The cramp is then said to be tonico-clonic. Occasionally, only myoclonias are present, somewhat reminding one of choreic movements.

In some cases the dyskinesia (= involuntary movements) of the upper limb is oscillatory and rythmical, resulting in tremor. Since this tremulation occurs only in connection with writing or is but mininal in other manual activities, it is called *primary writing tremor*. For instance, Ohye *et al.* (1982) reported the case of a right-handed male who at age 47 noticed that his hand tended to tremble when he wrote. At first, he could control the tremor by stiffening his arm. However, over the next three years the severity of the disorder gradually increased. The writing tremulation could no longer be controlled and the patient's script became illegible. All other manual activities involving the right hand remained undisturbed, though.

In a number of patients the tremor is elicited by the position taken by the wrist, hand or fingers when writing. For instance, Klawans *et al.* (1982) have reported cases in which sustained pronation of the wrist invariably resulted in shaking of the forearm. Since such pronation is necessary for writing, the act of writing was constantly hampered by the provoked tremor.

Sometimes, as in the second case described by Martinez-Martin and

Pareja (1984), dystonia, irregular jerks and tremor are all simultaneously present in attempts to write.

In a few cases, writing is impeded not by involuntary contractions but by a painless weakness of the fingers and hand which can no longer be made to perform writing movements. This form of writer's cramp then is a sort of writing impotence. It is sometimes called the paralytic form of writer's cramp, although the hand does not show the typical spasticity or flaccidity of paralyzed limbs.

Finally, patients may be encountered who complain that they can no longer properly control their hand when writing. They feel no pain, their muscles are not unduly contracted, there is no real dyskinesia, but their hand writes precipitously and illegibly and the patients seem to be unable to do anything about it.

2.2. *Progressive or Instantaneous Difficulty*

In a number of cases, the disorder of graphomotricity manifests itself after the patient has been writing for some time, that is to say that the disturbance comes about slowly and does not prevent the patient from writing a few lines or even a few paragraphs.

In other cases, on the contrary, the impediment appears as soon as the patient starts writing, preventing him from forming more than just a few words. In extreme cases, not a single word can be written in full. These patients are unable to sign their name.

Sometimes, as in the case reported by Alajouanine *et al.* (1928), an evolution can be observed: the cramp, which at first occurred after the patient had been writing for a certain time, now comes about after a few seconds or as soon as the patient picks up his pen.

At times, the affection sets in insidiously, the patient experiencing at first writing difficulties only when tired or tensed. In other cases, the disorder begins suddenly, the patient discovering to his surprise that he has become unable to write legibly or without pain.

The impediment is not always permanent. For instance, a patient of Ravits and coworkers (1985) had had symptom-free intervals of up to two years.

2.3. *Writing Posture*

Many patients with writer's cramp hold their pen or pencil in an unusual manner. This abnormal grip may be observed as soon as the subject grasps the pen(cil) or, on the contrary, appear slowly as the act of writing progresses. S.D., one of Crisp and Moldofsky's patients (1965) altered his tight grip in various ways during writing so that finally the pen would be held between the thumb and fifth finger. Other patients (e.g., Gowers,

1868, vol. 2, p. 662) hold their pen between index and middle fingers. One of our own patients used his thumb and index finger, while the other fingers rested in extended position on the page.

Some patients constantly drop their pen(cil) or find it necessary to readjust their grip on it. A few of them use a special pen(cil) provided with rings encircling their fingers, in order to stabilize their grip.

The overall writing posture may also be peculiar. For instance, a patient of Crisp and Moldofsky (1965) held his elbow elevated above the table and pressed his wrist firmly on the paper. A patient of Callewaert (1927) wrote with his arm pressed against his flank.

Some patients with writing tremor attempt to reduce the tremulation of their writing hand by steadying it with the other hand. Others who have cramp without tremor, may use a finger of their left hand to push their right hand along the line.

2.4. *Script*

Most of the time the script produced by those patients who can still write is erratic and after a few lines tends to become illegible. Not infrequently, the strokes testify to an excessive pressure exerted on the pen(cil). Indeed, the paper may be perforated at places.

2.5. *Unusual Writing Techniques*

In writer's cramp, changing one's ordinary way of writing may have — at least temporarily — a beneficial influence on one's performance. It is commonly observed during examination that patients, even those with an instantaneous cramp, are able to write if they are given an unusually thick pencil, or are requested to write with a piece of chalk on a blackboard, to hold their pen(cil) like a dagger in a closed fist, or to write with their index finger after they have dipped it in ink.

A number of patients spontaneously adopt special writing techniques which enable them to write at least a few lines. For instance, a patient of Alajouanine *et al.* (1928) found that using a pencil instead of a pen enabled him to make short jottings.

However, the effect of these tricks tend to wear off. Ultimately Alajouanine *et al.*'s patient had nearly as much difficulty in using a pencil as in using a pen. He then found another expedient: if he did not rest his forearm on the table, he could still form a few words.

The use of unaccustomed writing techniques may result in strange postures of fingers, hand, arm and/or trunk. Some clinicians feel that these abnormal positions, even though they may temporarily render writing less arduous, in the long run add to the patient's impairment.

2.6. *The Other Hand*

Not infrequently patients afflicted with writer's cramp teach themselves to write with their other hand. In a number of cases, this shift is easy, as the patients are left-handers who have been taught (sometimes forcibly) at school to write with their right hand and have used this hand for writing ever since.

Patients who resort to the nonaffected hand may after some time experience writing difficulties in that hand also. In other words, the impediment may become bilateral.

One of Poore's patients (1897, p. 65), who was afflicted with severe writer's cramp on the right, taught himself to write with the left hand. However, when writing with that hand he could not help "making spiderlike movements with the fingers of the right".

2.7. *Other Unimanual Activities*

Writer's cramp is, by definition, a selective impairment of writing. However, with the passing of time, the inability may extend to other unimanual activities. For instance, in the case reported by Ravits *et al.* (1985), involuntary supination of the forearm came about at first only when the patient engaged in writing. Later, other activities such as typing, playing the piano or the guitar, serving or dealing cards, were similarly disturbed. Of the 11 patients examined by Hughes and McLellan (1985),

only four had simple writer's cramp. The other seven noticed slight difficulty with a small number of other activities, the commonest being using a knife and fork and stirring tea with a spoon. However, in only two of the subjects were these other functions regarded as a significant level of disability, in contrast to the disability conferred by their writer's cramp.

At times, however, simple writer's cramp remains remarkably stable, leaving all other unimanual activities unaffected, with the possible exception of detailed drawing. For instance, Martinez-Martin and Pareja (1984) reported the case of a 70-year-old lawyer who had been suffering from writer's cramp for 35 years. His disorder was severe, his script being barely legible. None the less, the patient had for years been practising artistic painting without problems except for the drawing of small details. He used his typewriter for written communication.

Sheehy and Marsden (1982) have coined the phrase *dystonic writer's cramp* to refer to cases in which the cramp is not simple, i.e., in which other skilled manual activities are disturbed in addition to writing. In a group of 29 patients with writer's cramp, these authors found 8 who had had so-called dystonic writer's cramp from the beginning of their illness, another 8 who had simple writer's cramp initially but later developed features of dystonic writer's cramp (Sheehy and Marsden call this type of cramp *progressive writer's cramp*), and finally 13 who had had simple writer's cramp since the onset of their disorder.

2.8. *Concomitant Deficits*

Not infrequently, patients with writer's cramp evidence on examination one or more subtle neurological symptoms. The most frequent concomitant sign is a slight postural or intention tremor of the upper extremities. This tremor may be bilateral or limited to the side with writer's cramp. The affected limb may also show dystonic posture either spontaneously (when the patient sits or walks) or induced by rapid movements. There may be loss of arm swing on the affected side (when the patient walks) and minimal increase in muscle tone.

In a number of cases, writer's cramp remains for some years the only symptom, then a more or less complex neurological symptomatology progressively develops. For instance, Alajouanine *et al.* (1926) reported the case of a man who at age 32 started to suffer from monosymptomatic writer's cramp. About 10 years later spasmodic torticollis with involuntary rotation of the head to the right appeared. This was accompanied by involuntary gyration of the body to the right, without fall. This latter symptom spontaneously cleared after two weeks, while left neurotomy could improve the torticollis. About 20 years later, involuntary movements somewhat reminiscent of chorea appeared in the head and neck, and to a lesser extent also in the two upper limbs. The oro-pharyngeal dyskinesia caused dysarthria and dysphagia, while the dyskinesia of the upper limbs impeded writing.

A number of patients with writer's cramp complain of intermittent pain in the shoulder or in the neck. This pain may be experienced even when they are not writing. Objective signs of cervicarthrosis are sometimes found radiologically.

Occasionally, a slight reduction of muscle strength is observed in the affected hand. Muscle wasting seems to be extremely rare.

2.9. *Occupational Cramp*

Many patients with writer's cramp are people whose professional activities entail much writing. For instance, Poore (1897) had a patient, a clerk, who "did, on an average, nine hours' writing a day". Another patient of his had done "an immense amount of writing during the last thirteen years, often writing 'against time' ". A patient of Alajouanine *et al.* (1928) was a clerk in a military office. His job entailed "de longues écritures" (long writing duties). The patient treated by Moldofsky (1971) started to suffer from writer's cramp soon after he had been promoted to a position involving "much unaccustomed writing". Five of Crisp and Moldofsky's seven patients (1965) had occupations involving a considerable amount of writing. And 12 of Sheehy and Marsden's 29 patients (1985) had clerical duties while another five had accountancy as their vocation. Only five had jobs, like hairdressing, which did not involve extensive writing. Writer's cramp, then, appears to be to a large extent an occupational cramp. Pai (1947) disagreed with this view, pointing out that only a minority of his patients were clerical workers. However, his criteria for including patients with writer's cramp were very loose and it is not at all sure that all of his patients, who were army recruits, actually suffered from the disease discussed here. As a consequence, Pai's cases can hardly be used to reject the notion that writer's cramp occurs primarily in people who have to do a lot of writing professionally.

Interestingly, the disorder is but rarely observed in schoolchildren, despite the extensive writing which some of them, especially high school pupils, have to do. In fact, the affection typically begins between the ages of 20 and 50. In three of the few reported cases of children with writer's cramp (André-Thomas, 1952; Klawans *et al.*, 1982), there was evidence of perinatal brain damage.

2.10. *Premorbid Penmanship*

Anamnestically a number of patients with writer's cramp appear to have had fine handwriting and to have valued calligraphy. For instance, a patient of Poore's (1897) was a writing clerk who "wrote an excellent hand (. . .). By reason of his neat style he was constantly employed in copying balance-sheets." One of our own patients, Jean B., reported that as a pupil and as a student he always wanted to have well-written neat note-books. He would use a fountain-pen rather than a ball-pen because he felt that he could write more elegantly with a fountain-pen. Another of our cases, Rosy B., proudly showed us her school note-books, which she had preserved because, she said, they were so clean and so clearly written. A patient of Callewaert's (1927) won a prize in a calligraphy contest.

Other patients on the contrary found the acquisition of a legible, well-formed script difficult. One of our patients, Felix H., who was left-handed, was taught at school to write with his right hand. As a pupil he wrote more slowly and with less facility than his classmates. When he had to hurry, his handwriting degenerated into a scribble.

2.11. *Shame*

Some patients with writer's cramp are ashamed of their writing problem and do everything they can to conceal it from their relatives, friends and colleagues. They carefully avoid writing in the presence of others. sometimes forging odd excuses for not using written language. A patient of

Callewaert's (1927), who was a notary, reported that he endeavoured to conceal his impairment in all possible ways and that he could never write with someone present.

Other patients, while they do not really try to keep their affliction secret, are inclined to play it down. For instance, Crisp and Moldofsky (1965) say of their seven patients that "they were mostly concerned to minimize their writing difficulty to others".

One of the reasons why some patients with writer's cramp avoid writing when other people are present, may be that their writing difficulties increase when they are being watched. As a matter of fact, sufferers from writer's cramp not infrequently indicate that they can write for a longer period of time or with less difficulty if they are alone.

2.12. *Sex Ratio*

Gowers in 1888 indicated that writer's cramp was "very much more common in males than in females". In 1969, Brain's handbook (p. 1007) still noted that "both sexes are affected, but males more often than females". It is not clear, however, whether the higher incidence of the disease in the male sex is genetically or socially determined. Since mogigraphia is an occupational cramp, it is natural that in the past there should have been more males than females affected, as men engaged in extensive professional writing far more often than women. Nowadays, with both sexes becoming equal in matters of vocational activities, the sex ratio may be approaching 1:1, unless, of course, writer's cramp is one of those numerous diseases that affect males more than females regardless of social environment.

3.1. PATHOGENESIS

3.1. *Organogenic vs. Psychogenic Impediment*

The etiology of writer's cramp has been a much-disputed issue ever since the condition started to be studied. Basically, two views oppose each other. A number of clinicians hold writer's cramp to be organic in nature. For instance, Barré (1952) was convinced that "la crampe des écrivains est bien une affection organique" (writer's cramp is really an organic disease). Sheehy and Marsden (1982) concur that "writer's cramp is a physical illness".

Others, on the contrary, deny that the condition results from a specific lesion of the central or peripheral nervous system and regard writer's cramp as a form of neurosis. For instance, Luchsinger and Arnold (1970, II, p. 775) claimed that the impediment was a *Beschäftigungsneurose*, i.e., an occupational neurosis. In Oken's opinion (1970, p. 740) writer's cramp is a psychiatric problem and "its psychogenic nature is evident".

Who in this controversy is right? Is writer's cramp organic or functional? Is it caused by a lesion or disease of the central nervous system or is it the somatization of a psychological problem?

It would seem that in a number of cases the organic origin of the disorder can hardly be doubted. For instance, Siegfried et al. (1969) have reported on a patient who evidenced a slight intention tremor of both hands in some manual activities. As soon as he attempted to write, however, the tremor was so pronounced that only illegible scribble could be produced. Drawing was similarly impaired. Electrocoagulation of the nucleus ventralis lateralis of the left thalamus significantly improved the patient's writing by reducing the intention tremor. Stereotactic thalamotomy performed by Ohye et al. (1982) on three patients with primary writing tremor also put an end to the disorder of graphomotricity. In cases like these, where selective electric coagulation of parts of the basal ganglia relieve the symptoms, there is little reason to doubt the organic origin of the writing impediment.

The organicity of the ailment also seems demonstrated in those cases which can be influenced by drugs known to have an action on the basal ganglia. For instance, in two patients with primary writing tremor, Klawans et al. (1982) found that injection of anticholinergics resulted in marked improvement of the writing performance. There was prompt reversal of the improvement after injection of a cholinergic agent.

This report and the papers by Siegfried et al. (1969) and Ohye et al. (1982) point to the extrapyramidal system as responsible for writing tremor when the condition has a central organic origin.

However, not only lesions of the central but also lesions of the peripheral nervous system can bring about writer's cramp. For instance, Péron et al. (1951) reported a case in which on examination a particular point was discovered in the scaphoid region which was very sensitive to pressure. Infiltration of the region with procaine noticeably improved the graphospasm. In this case, then, peripheral neuralgia seems to have been the cause of the writing problem.

Several instances of writer's cramp following damage to one or more of the arm nerves were reported by Poore (1897) at the end of the last century. And Barré in 1925 described a patient in whom writer's cramp was associated with, and probably caused by, cervical osteo-arthritis (cervicarthrosis).

In cases where writer's cramp can be shown, or may safely be assumed, to have an organic origin, it is to be presumed that not only writing but also other skilled (uni)manual activities are disturbed. As a matter of fact, Hughes and McLellan (1985) studying electromyographically the intensity of contraction in the flexor and extensor muscles of the fingers and forearm during the performance of a series of writing and nonwriting tasks by 11 right-handed patients suffering from writer's cramp and by a group of matched controls, found that the patients had "highly significant increases in muscle activation especially in the triceps muscle which was overactive in all but one of the tasks" (namely drawing). This observation suggests that in patients with writer's cramp, the disorder of motor control is not confined to writing but extends to other unimanual activities as well. That the patients should complain primarily, and in some cases even exclusively, of a writing impediment is probably due to the fact that writing is often a sustained activity, pursued sometimes for hours on end. Other activities, like turning door-knobs or stirring tea with a spoon are of very short duration. They also require less skill. It is conceivable therefore that the patients are less aware of abnormal muscle contractions during the performance of relatively simple actions of short duration than during performance of a complex and long-lasting action. Understandably, people who instead of writing are in the habit of performing another skilled action for hours on end may develop the corresponding occupational cramp, e.g., violinist's cramp.

However, not in every case of writer's cramp can a lesion of the central or peripheral nervous system be demonstrated. The question then arises whether in patients without concomitant neurological symptoms the cramp might not be psychogenic. According to Brain (1969, p. 1007), when the patient has not other complaint than his writing problem and neurological examination is completely normal, writer's cramp should be considered psychogenic. In fact, Brain reasoned, neurologists do not know of any organic disorder in which movements are impaired only when they are components of one specific activity but remain unaffected in all other cases. Brain further found that writer's cramp affects both prime movers and their antagonists and thus resembles hysterical paralysis.

Patients with writer's cramp as their only symptom are sometimes considered to have feelings of anger but to be reluctant to discharge them. Since a clenched fist is often a psychobiological concomitant of the expression of anger, these patients view the more or less clenched posture of their hand in writing as a manifestation of the feelings they seek to repress. As a consequence, they experience difficulty in maintaining this posture and in continuing to write. In this view, then, writer's cramp is a conversion neurosis.

Some psychiatrists agree that writer's cramp is the bodily manifestation of a psychologic conflict but insist that this conflict may be different in different patients. In other words, writer's cramp may result from various psychic problems.

Other clinicians have expressed the view that writer's cramp is, in fact, a complex disturbance comprising both organic and psychic components.

André-Thomas and Ajuriaguerra (1943), for instance, have submitted that initially writer's cramp results from fatigue of the neuronal circuits involved in graphomotor activity. If the subject becomes concerned about his deficiency, his anxiety reflects negatively on his writing impediment, which tends to increase. This in turn augments the patient's anxiety and a vicious circle is created. In other words, a temporary and fairly moderate dysfunction tends to worsen and to become permanent under the influence of the psychic stress which it generates.

If fatigue is, in some cases at least, the prime mover of writer's cramp, what causes it? An obvious answer is: excessive writing. In this connection it is probably significant that the majority of sufferers from writer's cramp have vocations implying much writing.

However, not only the quantity of writing but also the quality of the written output may conceivably play a role in the occurrence of fatigue. If one applies oneself to producing handsome, calligraphic script, one may also overtrax the neuronal circuits involved in writing. And a number of patients with writer's cramp do report that they liked to write neatly.

Other individuals who may be thought to be susceptible to writing fatigue are left-handers who have been compelled to write with their non-preferred hand. In these people, writing may be a somewhat strenuous action requiring more neuromuscular effort than writing with the preferred hand. In this connection, it may be recalled that Poore (1897), who examined dozens of patients with writer's cramp, found among them an unusual proportion of left-handers who had been taught to write with their right hand. Two of our own patients, Felix H. and Pierre H., were also left-handers who in school learnt to write with their right hand.

Again, writing movements are probably among the most complex skilled movements man ever learns to perform. It takes the schoolchild years to acquire a quick, supple and legible hand. Therefore, the neuronal circuits subserving writing must be both multiple and delicate. If these circuits are strained either as a consequence of prolonged calligraphic writing or of writing with the nonpreferred hand, they may conceivably break down when the individual is put under psychological stress.

If this assumption is correct, what kind of stress is likely to precipitate writer's cramp? Gowers in 1888 noted that "many patients at the time of the onset of their affection, were enduring anxiety from family trouble, business worry, or weighty responsibilities". It would seem that one of the family troubles which can trigger off writer's cramp is the loss of a cherished relative. For instance, two of Crisp and Moldofsky's seven patients (1965) "had suffered the loss of a parent immediately preceding the development of their writer's cramp". One of the 29 patients examined by Sheehy and Marsden (1982) "reported writing difficulty soon after the death of a parent" and another "described the dramatic onset of a jerking dystonic writers' cramp when trying to write the members of his family and tell them of his son's sudden death". One of our own patients started to have writing difficulty soon after her husband had died in a fire.

Business worries, on the other hand, were reported by several of Crisp and Moldofsky's patients as well as by some of our own patients. As for the weight of professional responsibilities, it was present in two of Crisp and Moldofsky's seven cases and in two of our own patients (Felix H., Lucien J.). These four patients appeared to be conscientious, indeed meticulous workers, eager to please their superiors.

None the less, as a group, patients with writer's cramp do not appear prone to neuroticism. For instance, in Sheehy and Marsden's group of 29 patients (1985) the incidence of psychiatric symptoms was not greater than in the population at large. As for Crisp and Moldofsky (1965), they felt that their patients "were particularly tense, striving, sensitive, conscientious, precise, emotionally overcontrolled people with a need to help others and with a tendency to become overdependent in their interpersonal relationships and work". However, none of them was found to have a hysterical or neurotic personality.

It would appear, then, that psychological stress may act as the trigger mechanism in writer's cramp, by upsetting the fragile homeostasis of a complex cerebral network that subserves graphomotricity and that for some genetic or maturational reason happens to be less robust than in other individuals. In other words, the weak physiological point becomes the breaking point when the subject experiences psychical difficulties.

4. THERAPY

Opinions vary not only as regards the etiopathology of writer's cramp but also as regards the possibility to treat it. For instance, André-Thomas and Ajuriaguerra (1943) upheld the view that the disease could hardly be remedied. Callewaert (1927) was less pessimistic. He claimed that people with writer's cramp could be successfully treated if their writing impediment was due to a faulty regulation of physiological tonus resulting in muscular overcontraction and lack of muscular coordination. Such functional stuttering of the hand, as he called it, could be improved by teaching patients a new graphomotor style including supple finger and hand movements, a slightly flexed wrist position and a slanted handwriting. Relaxation therapy and control of tonus in nonwriting hand and finger movements should precede the acquisition of the new style (Callewaert, 1937).

Interestingly, as early as 1877, Gowers made writing mode the primary cause of writer's cramp. If the displacement of the pen along the line is effected by the muscles of the fingers and hand, this may, according to Gowers, easily result in overcontraction of these muscles and hence cause writer's cramp. Far better is it "to write from the shoulder", that is to say to rest one's forearm, wrist and little finger gently on the table and to move the writing limb along the line using the muscles of the shoulder. Gowers was of the opinion that "if all persons wrote from the shoulder, writer's cramp would practically cease". Accordingly, he recommended that this mode of writing should be systematically taught at school. Prevention of writer's cramp, he concluded, rests not with doctors but with teachers.

Girard (1949) shared the view that writer's cramp is a stammer of the hand. Indeed, he stated that stuttering is the exact equivalent of writer's cramp in spoken language. According to Girard, the two impediments, have in fact the same origin: a lack of cerebral dominance. All stutterers and all patients with writer's cramp are shifted left-handers, in whom both hemispheres compete as soon as speech or writing is performed in an automatic way. This rivalry results in antagonistic muscle contractions which prevent the subject from proceeding with speaking or writing. Accordingly, stuttering and writer's cramp would cease to exist if left-handed children were no longer compelled to use their nonpreferred hand. Girard therefore agreed with Gowers that the prophylaxis of writer's cramp rests with parents and teachers.

It is strange that neither Callewaert nor Girard should have been struck by the fairly obvious difference that exist between stuttering and writer's cramp. While most stutterers do experience blocks which may in a way be compared with graphospasms in sufferers from writer's cramp, they also make repetitions and sound prolongations, which have no equivalents in mogigraphia. Moreover, few stutterers complain that their blocks are painful, while writer's cramp often is. Again, despite their blocks, repetitions and sound prolongations, most stutterers are able to speak, whereas quite a number of people with writer's cramp cannot write more than a few words. Also, stutterers often evidence synkinesias, i.e., concomitant involuntary contractions of muscles of the face, limbs or trunk, resulting in such movements as eye blinking, sniffing, stamping, etc. Such synkinesias have not been reported in patients with writer's cramp.

Last but not least, stuttering usually begins in childhood, whereas writer's cramp is rare in children. Indeed, adult stutterers do not seem to be more liable to writer's cramp than fluent speakers, which should be the case if the two diseases really had a common origin.

Yet, stuttering and writer's cramp do have a few features in common. Both are impediments that selectively affect a communicative activity. Oral activities such as eating, drinking, smoking, whistling and even singing are usually performed easily by stutterers, just as sufferers from writer's cramp have, at least initially, no difficulty in performing nonwriting manual activities with their affected hand. Moreover, stuttering ordinarily decreases and may even disappear temporarily when the stutterer is asked to speak in an unusual way, e.g., when he protracts his vowels, deliberately imitates a regional accent, or whispers. Similarly, writer's cramp generally fails to appear when the patient adopts an unusual mode of writing, such as writing with a piece of chalk on a blackboard.

Thus, there are similarities between stuttering and writer's cramp but they are outweighed by the differences. It is therefore doubtful whether the two conditions have a common etiology. As a matter of fact, the notion that communicative disorders such as stuttering (Travis, 1978), dyslexia (Orton, 1928) and writer's cramp (Girard, 1949) are due to insufficient cerebral dominance for language has never been proved.

Accordingly, other clinicians have used different therapeutical approaches. For instance, Liversedge and Sylvester (1955) reported some success with avoidance conditioning therapy. The patient wrote with an electrified pen which delivered electric shocks whenever it was excessively gripped or whenever it deviated from a prescribed course of lined patterns. Obviously, this method can only be used with patients suffering from psychogenic writer's cramp. Moreover, the treatment may cure the symptom but not its cause. Indeed, like all other punishment therapies, it may have negative effects on the patients.

Some have used psychoanalysis with patients suffering from writer's cramp, but the results do not appear very convincing.

As a matter of fact, writer's cramp, like stuttering, seems to be a disease that can have various origins ranging from the purely organic to the purely psychogenic with several intermediate stages. It is therefore desirable to study each case thoroughly and to try to ascertain the causal factor or factors in each individual patient. Obviously, most of the time, only a well-integrated clinical team comprising a neurologist, a neurophysiologist, a neurosurgeon, a neurolinguist or neuropsychologist and a psychiatrist will be able to carry out such a task. Only after each case has been carefully assessed can a therapy be devised that is likely to achieve if not a complete cure at least a durable improvement of the condition.

5. CONCLUSIONS

Writer's cramp, then, is a variegated disorder of graphomotricity that afflicts primarily people who have to do much professional writing. It is usually unilateral but may become bilateral after the patient has for some time used his nonaffected hand for writing. It can be, at least temporarily, relieved by resorting to an unusual writing mode. It may remain strictly confined to the act of writing or may eventually affect a number of nonwriting tasks as well. Its pathogenesis is still obscure. Probably it is purely neurogenic in some cases, purely psychogenic in others, and mixed in still others. Accordingly, each case has to be carefully investigated preferably by a multidisciplinary team, and an individual therapy has to be tailored in accordance with the team's findings.

REFERENCES

Alajouanine, T., Thurel, R. and Gopcevitch, X.: 1928, 'Syndrome choréique chronique à topographie brachio-cervico-faciale avec dysarthrie de type wilsonien, précédé, il y a trente ans, d'une crampe des écrivains et il y a vingt ans, d'un torticolis spasmodique', *Revue Neurologique* **35**, 530—540.

Barré, J.: 1925, 'Crampe des écrivains et arthrite cervicale', *Revue Neurologique* **32**, 651—652.

Barré, J.: 1952, 'La crampe des écrivains, maladie organique, ses formes, ses causes', *Revue Neurologique* **86**, 730.

Brain, R.: 1969, *Diseases of the Nervous System* (7th edn, rev. by J. Walton), Oxford University Press, London.

Callewaert, H.: 1927, 'Pathogénie de la crampe des écrivains. Epreuve de la rééducation', *Journal de Neurologie et de Psychiatrie* **27**, 371—377.

Callewaert, H.: 1937, 'Crampes professionnelles. Pathogénie. Formes cliniques. Traitement', *Le Scalpel* **90**, 1151—1167.

Crisp, A. and Moldofsky, H.: 1965, 'A psychosomatic study of writer's cramp', *British Journal of Psychiatry* **111**, 841—858.

Girard, P.: 1949, 'Les crampes fonctionnelles', in *Traité de médecine*, Pt. 16, Masson, Paris, pp. 1191—1197.

Gowers, W.: 1877, 'Writer's cramp', *Medical Times and Gazette* **2**, 536—538.

Gowers, W.: 1888, *A Manual of Diseases of the Nervous System*, Churchill, London.

Hughes, M. and McLellan, D.: 1985, 'Increased co-activation of the upper limb muscles in writer's cramp', *Journal of Neurology, Neurosurgery, and Psychiatry* **48**, 782—787.

Klawans, H., Glantz, R., Tanner, C. and Goetz, C.: 1982, 'Primary writing tremor: A selective action tremor', *Neurology* **32**, 203—205.

Liversedge, L. and Sylvester, J.: 1955, 'Conditioning techniques in the treatment of writer's cramp', *Lancet* **1**, 1147—1149.

Luchsinger, R. and Arnold, G.: 1970, *Handbuch der Stimm- und Sprachheilkunde*, Springer Verlag, Wien.

Martinez-Martin, P. and Pareja, F.: 1985, 'Familial writer's cramp', *Journal of Neurology, Neurosurgery, and Psychiatry* **48**, 487.

Moldofsky, H.: 1971, 'Occupational cramp', *Journal of Psychosomatic Research* **15**, 439—444.

Ohye, C., Miyazaki, M., Hirai, T., Shibazaki, T., Nakajima, H. and Nagaseki, Y.: 1982, 'Primary writing tremor treated by stereotactic selective thalamotomy', *Journal of Neurology, Neurosurgery, and Psychiatry* **45**, 988—997.

Oken, D.: 1970, 'Musculoskeletal disorders', in Arieti, S. (ed.), *American Handbook of Psychiatry*, Vol. 4, Pt. 2, Basic Books, New York, pp. 726—766.

Orton, S.: 1928, 'A physiological theory of reading disability and stuttering in children', *New England Journal of Medicine* **9**, 97—113.

Pai, M.: 1947, 'The nature and treatment of writer's cramp', *The Journal of Mental Science* **93**, 68—81.

Péron, N., Tardieu, G. and Cathala, H.: 1951, 'Crampe des écrivains et déterminations ostéo-articulaires du membre supérieur. Intérêt des infiltrations procaïniques locales', *Revue Neurologique* **84**, 57—59.

Poore, G.: 1897, *Nervous Affections of the Hand and Other Clinical Studies*, Smith, Elder and Co., London.

Ravits, J., Hallett, M., Baker, M. and Wilkins, D.: 1985, 'Primary writing tremor and myoclinic writer's cramp', *Neurology* **35**, 1387—1391.

Sheehy, M. and Marsden, C.: 1982, 'Writer's cramp: A focal dystonia', *Brain* **105**, 461—480.

Siegfried, J., Crowell, R. and Perret, E.: 1969, 'Cure of tremulous writer's cramp by stereotaxic thalamotomy', *Journal of Neurosurgery* **30**, 182—185.

Thomas, A.: 1952, 'Un cas de dysgraphie précoce. Hémorragie méningée à la naissance', *Revue Neurologique* **86**, 250—255.

Thomas, A. and Ajuriaguerra, J.: 1943, 'La crampe des écrivains est-elle une affection organique?', *La Presse Médicale* **26**, 376—377.

Travis, L.: 1978, 'The cerebral dominance theory of stuttering: 1931—1978', *Journal of Speech and Hearing Disorders* **43**, 278—281.

J. RISPENS AND I. A. VAN BERCKELAER

HYPERLEXIA: DEFINITION AND CRITERION

1. INTRODUCTION

Hyperlexia refers to a condition in which developmentally disordered children have advanced word recognition skills but show little reading comprehension. Clinicians have long been aware of the existence of such advanced, but specific and isolated abilities in mentally disordered children. Scheerer, Rothmann and Goldstein (1945) described a case of what they called an "idiot savant": an 11-year-old boy who, notwithstanding his behavioral problems and developmental delay, had an unusual skill in calendar computation and astonishing musical abilities. At the age of five he learned the letters from his toy blocks and developed subsequently good word recognition skills, but his comprehension remained poor. In other studies of such cases (Cain, 1969), advanced word recognition skills in the absence of comprehension have often been reported. In 1967 Silberberg and Silberberg coined the term hyperlexia to refer to this phenomenon. Several studies (Huttenlocher and Huttenlocher, 1973; Cobrinik, 1974, 1982; Elliott and Needleman, 1976; Richman and Kitchell, 1981; Healy, 1982; Needleman, 1984; Goldber and Rothermel, 1984; Frith and Snowling, 1983; Whitehouse and Harris, 1984; Siegel, 1984; Snowling and Frith, 1986; Healy and Aram, 1986) have documented the existence of the condition called hyperlexia.

However, a closer look at this literature reveals a number of inconsistencies, involving even the definition of the condition. In fact it can easily be demonstrated that researchers disagree on almost all important issues. Several authors (De Hirsch, 1971; Benton, 1978) conceive of hyperlexia as one of the subtypes of dyslexia; others (Healy, 1982; Needleman, 1982) state that hyperlexia is a specific syndrome, while Graziani, et al. (1983) conclude that hyperlexia is a nonspecific finding. Some studies (Whitehouse and Harris, 1984) suggest that hyperlexia is closely related to autism. However, Snowling and Frith (1986) conclude from their data that hyperlexia is not syndrome specific. In the same study a new criterion to classify children as truly hyperlexic was proposed.

It is tempting to conclude from this lack of consensus that the idea of the existence of a separate condition called hyperlexia should be discarded. At the same time it cannot be denied that apparently some children learn to read (often without formal instruction) on a level far ahead of their semantic skills. This is of course an intriguing phenomenon, which needs further attention.

R. M. Joshi (ed.), Written Language Disorders, 143—163.
© 1991 *Kluwer Academic Publishers. Printed in the Netherlands.*

It could have some advantage, at least for the sake of brevity, to classify those children as hyperlexic. But then it has to be clear what this term means. Further clarification of the concept of hyperlexia is therefore needed.

The purpose of this chapter is twofold. In the first part of the chapter we sketch briefly the state of the art of hyperlexia research and review the existing hyperlexia literature.

In the second part of the chapter we discuss in some detail a topic that is important for a proper understanding of hyperlexia. Our analysis of the literature demonstrates that until now the development of diagnostic criteria has been neglected. As a consequence, it is often obscure why a child in a particular study has been classified as hyperlexic. Several authors (Graziani et al., 1983; Goldberg and Rothermel, 1984) have already concluded that diagnostic criteria have not been well established, but they do not suggest a solution to this problem. In this chapter we therefore pay attention to the problem of the operationalization of the concept of hyperlexia.

We assessed the reading performance of 32 autistic children. We demonstrate that the number of children identified as hyperlexic is dependent on the criteria applied. Establishing diagnostic criteria is therefore an important issue.

2. HYPERLEXIA: DEFINITION, NATURE AND CAUSES

2.1. *Introduction*

In this section we briefly review the literature on hyperlexia. We discuss the two main topics of the research until now: the definition of the condition, and in the second place the nature of hyperlexia (including the problem of syndrome specificity). We do not pay much attention to the conflicting views regarding the etiology we found in the literature. It is our opinion that those views are in fact no more than sheer speculations.

2.2. *The Definition of Hyperlexia*

In 1967, Silberberg and Silberberg introduced the term hyperlexia to refer to children with word recognition skills far above their general intellectual capacities. They presented data of more than 20 children manifesting this condition. In another paper (Silberberg and Silberberg, 1971) they described this sample in more detail and they presented some theoretical explanations, relating hyperlexia to dyslexia.

However, it has been known for a long time that some disordered children have isolated splinter abilities. The so called savant literature contains a number of case reports in which these children are described.

The study of Scheerer *et al.* (1945) is a fine example of an extensive clinical picture of an idiot savant. In studies of this kind advanced word recognition skills are considered as merely one of the specific abilities found in these children.

Silberberg and Silberberg did more than just to introduce a new term for an already well-known phenomenon. Their study introduced a shift in attention. They did not emphasize that hyperlexia has to do with severely disordered children, often described in the savant literature as psychotic (Cain, 1969) or as autistic (Goodman, 1972). Silberberg and Silberberg stated that: "The concept of hyperlexia suggests a continuum of word recognition skills which may exist separate and apart from general verbal functioning" (Silberberg and Silberberg, 1971, p. 41). In other words, Silberberg and Silberberg defined hyperlexia mainly in terms of a discrepancy between word recognition skills and general verbal functioning. Of course they noticed that more than half of the children of their sample were more or less severely disordered, but in their theoretical reflections they did not make much of this observation. They conceived of hyperlexia primarily as the counterpart of dyslexia. Dyslexia means reading performance below the expected level whereas in hyperlexia the reverse is the case. They suggested, that the numbers of children classified as hyperlexic or dyslexic are equal.

In this description hyperlexia has been dissociated from childhood disorders. As a consequence Niensted (1968) used the term just to refer to the often found discrepancy between word recognition and comprehension in normal readers.

Although the term hyperlexia has been adopted by almost everybody describing the phenomenon of advanced word recognition skills, only a few researchers define hyperlexia in the same vein as Silberberg and Silberberg or Niensted. Elliott and Needleman (1976) point to the fact that advanced word recognition ability occurs in both normal and disordered children. They suggest that the term hyperlexia ". . . be redefined as a remarkably accelerated ability to recognize written words, which may or may not occur along with truly pathological conditions . . ." (Elliott and Needleman, 1976, p. 340). The study of Richman and Kitchell (1981) is the only other example we know in which hyperlexia is defined as a word recognition ability far above the expected level without reference to developmental delay.

In most of the studies on hyperlexia this condition is associated with behavioral and developmental disorders. Mehegan and Dreifuss (1972) reported on hyperlexia found in 12 brain-damaged children. These children showed a lag in their development and behavioral abnormalities associated with the hyperkinesis syndrome. They had an outstanding reading ability but their reading made a peculiar, compulsive and ritualistic impression.

Huttenlocher and Huttenlocher (1973) described three children exhibiting hyperlexia against a background of intellectual impairment and apraxic disorders. The authors suggested that the behavioral problems of these children point to autism. All children learned to read at an early age without much parental help.

In his study of the performance of hyperlexic children on a task involving the ability to decipher incomplete words, Cobrinik (1982) used a sample consisting of 9 boys. All children had profound developmental arrests, with IQs ranging from 42 to 70, with a mean of 50. Most of the children could read before the age of 5, again without parental help or encouragement.

Siegel (1984) presented a case history of one hyperlexic girl with a serious developmental delay especially in language. At the age of 7 her word recognition score was in the 86th percentile, but she failed to answer most of the questions that were asked after she had read a paragraph.

In the study of Goldberg and Rothermel (1984) eight children participated, all with language delays but superior reading ability. All but one of the children had learned to read before the age of 5 with little or no formal instruction. It is interesting to note that Goldberg and Rothermel selected their sample from a group of autistic children whose parents believed that they displayed savant skills.

The 21 hyperlexic children included in the study of Graziani et al. (1983) manifested not only a discrepancy between word recognition and comprehension of at least two grade levels but also impaired language comprehension during pre-school age. They were referred to a neurology outpatient service because of their language and behavioral problems. What is interesting in this study is that the children were tested twice: initially at the age of 3 to $5\frac{1}{2}$ years and again in the school age period (6—15). This retesting revealed that 8 children with average WISR-R IQs no longer manifested language problems and their reading comprehension was age appropriate. Graziani et al. therefore concluded that some children have a good prognosis, despite their hyperlexia, language, and behavioral problems during the pre-school period.

A somewhat special position in hyperlexia research is occupied by a number of studies (Healy, 1982; Healy et al., 1982; Needleman, 1982; Whitehouse and Harris, 1984; Healy and Aram, 1986) which stress that hyperlexia is a separate syndrome. Characteristics of this syndrome are: the condition occurs in a developmentally disordered population; it has an early manifestation; reading develops in the absence of reading instruction; reading has a compulsive, ritualistic quality and word recognition is far better than expected.

In these studies hyperlexia is indeed often closely related to severe childhood disorders, mostly autism. In Needleman's study 6 out of the 9 participating children had been diagnosed as autistic. Harris and Whitehouse (1984) confined their study to autistic children. Their sample consisted of 20 children, comprising a subsample of the 52 cases identified as hyperlexic out of a group of 155 children diagnosed as autistic. These figures suggest that about 30% of the children with autism could be classified as hyperlexic. The authors therefore speculated that hyperlexics may constitute a subgroup of autistic children.

The children described by Healy (1982) manifested behavioral problems mostly associated with autism, like physical stereotypes, absence of interest in toys, inflexibility and problems relating to peers. Healy (1982) therefore concluded that hyperlexia is closely related to autism.

In a recent study Snowling and Frith (1986) made some interesting observations regarding the definition of hyperlexia. They concluded that not all handicapped childred showing excellent decoding skils merit the label hyperlexia. A number of autistic or otherwise mentally retarded children in their study were able to comprehend reading materials at a level according to their verbal and general intellectual capacity, whereas their word recognition skills were above this level. They suggest that ". . . *true hyperlexia* is manifested in terms of both (surprising) decoding success *and* (surprising) comprehension failure (the surprise being in relation to verbal ability)" (Snowling and Frith, 1986, p. 410; their italics). In other words they suggested hyperlexia should be defined in terms of a double discrepancy.

Another finding of Snowling and Frith is that hyperlexia is not syndrome specific. In their sample they could not find any relation between dyslexia and autism.

This brief review of the literature shows a number of differences in the description of the condition. One of the main issues has to do with the relation between hyperlexia and childhood disorders. Traditionally hyperlexia has been conceived as closely related to a developmentally disordered population. Anecdotal reports in clinical and savant literature hinting at the existence of the condition, established this tradition, which is continued in most of recent hyperlexia research. It is therefore partially a matter of convention or definition to associate hyperlexia with a disordered population. Dissociating hyperlexia from a disordered population has several consequences. Hyperlexia is conceived then as advanced word recognition skills compared with reading comprehension. The study of Niensted demonstrated that this is not an uncommon finding in normal children during the process of learning to read.

The moment hyperlexia is dissociated from a disordered population the question arises how it relates to dyslexia. We already sketched the position of Silberman and Silberman, who view hyperlexia as a counterpart of dyslexia. De Hirsch (1971) argues that hyperlexia in fact means poor reading and should therefore be regarded as a manifestation of dyslexia. Richman and Kitchell (1981) hold the same point of view. They state that the so-called superior reading performance of the hyperlexics is in fact no more than sight-word recognition. When comprehension and other language skills are considered it becomes apparent that hyperlexics are in fact poor readers. Benton (1976) suggests for that reason that hyperlexia has to be considered as one of the subtypes of dyslexia. Healy and Aram (1986), although stating that hyperlexia is closely associated with autism, point to a possible similarity with dyslexia because in both a genetic factor seems to be involved.

We therefore conclude that hyperlexia should be confined to a disordered population.

A second controversial issue concerns the question whether aspects such as early onset and the peculiar, compulsory character of the reading should be part of the definition. In most studies the presence of one or more of those elements is reported. Sometimes (e.g., Snowling and Frith, 1986) early onset and the ritualistic nature of the reading behavior is not mentioned.

2.3. *Diagnostic Criteria*

These differences in the description of the condition have far-reaching consequences when it comes to operationalization into a set of diagnostic criteria. Studies differ widely with respect to classification criteria that are applied. In a relatively small number of studies (Silberberg and Silberberg, 1971; Richman and Kitchell, 1982) the only criterion seems to be the single discrepancy between word recognition and IQ or another measurement of verbal skills or reading comprehension. Those authors who conceive of hyperlexia as a separate syndrome or stress the association with childhood disorders apply a number of criteria in addition to single discrepancy: early onset, no formal instruction, ritualistic character of the reading behavior. We already mentioned Snowling and Frith (1986) who suggested identification based on a double discrepancy.

Another problem arises when it comes to the measurement of a discrepancy. Most studies simply state the existence of a discrepancy, without further explaining the stability and significance of that discrepancy. In a number of studies the procedure described by Silberberg and Silberberg (1971) is applied. They suggested comparing actual and expected grade level: when the observed grade score exceeds the expected grade level the child is classified as hyperlexic, if the difference is 1.5 and more grades when the child is in Grade 1 or 2, and 2.0 or more grades when the child is in Grade 3 and up. They also suggested a procedure to meet the problem that most children participating in hyperlexia research are not in their age-appropriate grade while norm tables of most of the reading tests depend upon age. They therefore entered the table where the actual grade placement approximates IQ 100 on the table. Then the expected grade level, corresponding to the IQ of the child, is read out of the table.

This procedure has several weak points. A practical objection is that in norm tables of several reading tests no corresponding IQs are found. To solve this problem it is sometimes simply assumed that Grade 1 word recognition level corresponds with a mental age of 6—7 years (Graziani *et al.*, 1983). But even when reading score and IQ are given, the procedure has its inadequacies. The transformation of a reading score to a grade level score excludes the possibility of testing the significance of the difference in a statistically more sophisticated way. In the second place it must be noted that regression effects are neglected. Predicting grade level from an IQ without adjusting for regression effects, seems very risky (Willson and Reynolds, 1984). This holds especially in hyperlexia research, in which samples mostly include children with low IQs.

For all those reasons one cannot be sure that the studies we have reviewed would classify the same children as hyperlexic. In a number of studies (Graziani *et al.*, 1983; Snowling and Frith, 1986) this lack of diagnostic criteria has been noted.

A study of Epps *et al.* (1983) clearly demonstrates the relevance of adequate operationalization of the definition of a disorder. They studied the impact of different criteria on the number of children classified as learning disabled. They applied 14 different operationalizations of three categories of definitions of learning disability to the same group of children. Depending on the definition the percentage of children identified as learning disabled ranged from 5.3 to 69.6. The number of children identified as dyslexic depends on the operationalization of the definition of dyslexia into a number of diagnostic criteria.

The same holds true for hyperlexia research. Defining hyperlexia in terms of a double discrepancy would have far-reaching consequences for sampling procedures. For instance, of the 20 children participating in the Whitehouse and Harris (1984) study, only 5 would be identified as hyperlexic on the basis of a double discrepancy. In the next section we shall say more about the development of diagnostic criteria.

2.4. *The Nature of Hyperlexia*

The definitions we have reviewed thus far can hardly be regarded as very satisfying. They offer only a rather vague description of the condition without reference to the specific nature or the possible causes. However, this should not be a surprise, since the aim of most studies is limited to document the existence of hyperlexia. The studies (Cain, 1969; Mehegan and Dreifuss, 1972; Huttenlocher and Huttenlocher, 1973; Goodman, 1972) fitting into the savant tradition do not go into the details of the reading performance of the hyperlexics. In most cases scores on word recognition tests are mentioned and some remarks are made about reading comprehension, but no attempt is made to analyze more in detail the excellent word recognition performance with the help of reading theories.

This results in a rather straightforward view on the nature of hyperlexia. Huttenlocher and Huttenlocher (1973) believe that hyperlexics are unable to associate speech sounds (presented either in a written or in a spoken form) with meaning. They consider this as a basic language deficit resulting probably from a parietal lobe disorder. It is interesting to note that in recent research using an experimental procedure, this finding has been confirmed. Processing of meaning by ear or by eye does not make any difference, although both are considerably below age level (Snowling and Frith, 1986).

Healy (1982), Healy *et al.* (1982) and Healy and Aram (1986) pointed to the language problems of hyperlexic children. They state that hyperlexia means "... a genetically linked, neurologically-based impairment of basic systems of information processing, particularly affecting aspects of symbolic language ability" (Healy and Aram, 1986, p. 249).

In most studies (Mehegan and Dreifuss, 1972; Cain, 1969; Cobrinik, 1972) marked abnormalities in language and speech are indeed reported. Persistent echolalia and difficulties to comprehend instructions are often found. Very often there is a history of delayed speech development. Healy *et al.* (1982) suggested that language performance is below chronological age especially in language comprehension tests. Healy described in some detail reading performances of her sample of hyperlexics. She concluded that the reading problems of these children are on the level of sentences or connected discourse. Children gave the impression of not having grasped the meaning of what they had read, although they could sound out all the words in the text. She observed that intonation and expression were absent.

Different aspects of the reading performance of hyperlexics have been studied. Cobrinik (1982) compared the performance of hyperlexics and normal children on an incomplete word task, consisting of a series of 14 words degraded by means of deletion of identifying elements of the letters. The major aim of this study was to determine the capacity of hyperlexics to decipher the words compared with the performance of the controls. (The controls had significantly higher mean reading scores, compared to the hyperlexics. Data about the IQs of the controls are lacking; the IQs of the hyperlexics ranged from 42 to 70).

The hyperlexics performed better than the controls on this incomplete word task, suggesting a superior visual recognition capacity. Cobrinik was rather careful in the interpretation of this finding. He suggests that it may be possible to respond to simple word recognition tasks as if they were merely visual configurations. The fact that hyperlexics perform well on visual tasks offers an explanation for their relatively good word recognition skills. Visual recognition may be mediated by the right hemisphere. In a number of other studies good visual recognition performance has been reported.

Cobrinik offered a far from complete explanation for the word recognition performance. In this study no attention has been given to the syntactic or semantic proficiency of the hyperlexics. It is difficult to understand how hyperlexics are able to sound out nonsense words they have never seen before: good visual recognition alone may not be sufficient.

In her case report, Siegel (1984) pointed to the fact that the advanced word recognition skills of hyperlexics are the reverse of what is found in normal readers. In the process of learning to read most often semantic skills of the children tend to be ahead of their phonological capacity. She concludes from the fact that hyperlexics are able to read nonwords that they have adequate phonological skills. Her data (scores on different language tests) seem to suggest that semantic skills are lacking. This means that hyperlexics do recognize words using only a phonological route. However, we have to note that her data are not very specific as far as semantic impairment is concerned.

Frith and Snowling (1983) compared normal readers, dyslexics and autistic children, matched on reading age. A number of reading tasks were used, like normal words, nonsense words, abstract versus concrete words, a gap test.

They observed a striking difference between the reading performances of dyslexics and hyperlexics. The latter revealed a number of adequate linguistic competencies. Their phonological performance was age appropriate. Frith and Snowling concluded from the fact that effects like the abstract/concrete class word effect, influence of interference (measured by a Stroop-like test) were observed in the reading performance of hyperlexics in the same way as in normal readers, that a number of semantic aspects are intact in these children. They suggested that their reading problems are not on the word level.

This conclusion is also drawn by Goldberg and Rothermel (1984) in their study of the reading process of hyperlexic children. They used a great number of reading tasks (words, sentences, nonsense words) and reading related tasks (lexical decision tasks). There was no control group. Their data suggest that the problem of the reading of hyperlexics is in the domain of reading connected discourse. Many hyperlexic children exhibited extreme difficulties in reading paragraphs. Goldberg and Rothermel (as well as a number of other researchers) reported that several children show symptoms of distress when they are confronted with this kind of tasks. One did not respect white space between the words.

In a second study Snowling and Frith analyzed reading comprehension of hyperlexics (Snowling and Frith, 1986). Their sample consisted of 20 subjects of relatively high verbal ability and 20 children of low verbal ability. Both groups contained a number of normal, autistic and nonautistic but retarded children. (The groups were relatively small.) Several tasks were used, e.g., sentences containing homographs, presented in several conditions (at the beginning or at the end of the disambiguating context) texts of different lengths, with a cloze procedure.

The authors concluded that the performance of the autistic (hyperlexic) children could not be distinguished from that of the mildly retarded group. They therefore claimed that hyperlexia is not a syndrome-specific phenomenon.

More important is the finding that both the autistic and mildly retarded readers with high verbal capacity had a comprehension skill adequate to their verbal ability; they performed on the expected level (compared with their verbal capacity). For this reason these children cannot be diagnosed as hyperlexic, although their decoding skill is indeed above the expected level. This does not hold for the low-verbal-ability autistic group. They performed worse than their nonhandicapped controls with the same decoding skills. These children are therefore the true hyperlexics.

This failure to comprehend larger units of meaning in connected discourse cannot be attributed to poor general linguistic skill — although these are poor — because of the fact that hyperlexics perform below their expected level, nor is poor word knowledge the factor that causes this comprehension problem.

2.5. *Preliminary Conclusion*

The concept of hyperlexia has its roots in the so-called savant literature. Clinicians were struck by the advanced word recognition skills of these children. In a number of studies a more detailed picture of the condition has been sketched. The ease with which hyperlexic readers sound out words is indeed a striking feature. But they are not just "barking at printed words". Their word recognition is more than the ability to react to words as visual configuration. Hyperlexics are able to read nonsense words, and the interference effects found in normal reading do occur in hyperlexic reading as well.

The reading problems of a hyperlexic child have to do with the inability to understand connected discourse. What should be done in following studies of hyperlexia is to explain the nature of this failure. Word recognition need not bother us, but the apparent lack of comprehension of sentences and beyond should be investigated.

Our brief exposition of the literature has also demonstrated that progress in hyperlexia research is hampered by a number of unanswered questions — sometimes not even recognized as such. We demonstrated the existence of differences in defining the condition. We also found that diagnostic criteria have not been established. In the next section we shall discuss this topic more extensively.

3. THE DEVELOPMENT OF DIAGNOSTIC CRITERIA

3.1. *Introduction*

The aim of this section is to discuss in some detail one of the issues playing an important part in the development of diagnostic criteria, namely the meaurement of a discrepancy. Establishing diagnostic criteria depends to a great extent on the content and clarity of the definition of the condition. A common feature in all available definitions of hyperlexia is the idea of a discrepancy. A child is classified as hyperlexic if his actual word-recognition skill (Y_{obs}) is better than his expected reading score (Y_{exp}). Operationalization of this discrepancy between Y_{obs} and Y_{exp} constitutes the main problem in the process of developing diagnostic criteria. We shall discuss some of the problems involved and we investigate the effect of different decisions on the number of children identified as hyperlexic.

In the first place a decision has to be made about the predictor. The literature we reviewed offers a number of possible answers to this question: intelligence (verbal IQ, full-scale IQ), language competency (some language test), academic achievement (grade level), reading comprehension (some reading test) are used to predict the expected level of word recognition. Of course the definition of hyperlexia should answer the question which predictor has to be chosen. It is not our intention to discuss, from a theoretical point of view, which predictor should be preferred. However, it could be interesting to know whether different predictors yield different numbers of children classified as hyperlexic.

The same holds for the issue raised by Snowling and Frith (1986), suggesting that true hyperlexia implies a double discrepancy. The definition of hyperlexia should decide whether true hyperlexia implies the existence of a double discrepancy. Again, we want to investigate the impact of this choice on the number of children classified as hyperlexic.

In the second place a measurement is needed, prescribing how to predict the criterion (Y_{exp}) and how to test the significance of the difference between Y_{obs} and Y_{exp}. We shall discuss this problem in some detail here.

3.2. *Measurement Models*

For many years considerable attention has been paid to the problem of measuring a discrepancy. The professional literature on dyslexia contains a host of measurement models, prescribing how to measure a discrepancy. Some are not so much models, but (rather cryptic) formulas, or rules of thumb, stemming from clinical practice.

We shall not go into detail by describing and evaluating all the models that could be used. To start with we exclude all procedures that lack sufficient theoretical, empirical or psychometric justification. Two broad categories of measurement procedures remain. In the first group (in dyslexia research known as the "two years behind grade level" model) scores on tests of academic achievement are transformed into the corresponding grade levels and then compared to the average grade score of children with the same amount of reading instruction. If the difference is more than two years (or 20 months) the difference is considered to be important.

Box 1 depicts this model and several of its variants.

BOX 1

Model 1   *Reading age discrepancy model*

ERA − RA ⩾ 20 months

ERA (Expected Reading Age) = expected score on reading test, based on number of months of reading instruction, corresponding with 5th decile of age group.

RA   (Reading Age) = observed reading score, expressed as grade level.

Variants

(a) Cumulative discrepancy, for example,
          Grade 1:   8 months
          Grade 2: 14 months
          Grade 3: 20 months, etc.

(b) Discrepancy with IQ Restriction, for example,
          the model is applied if IQ ⩾ 85.

In this procedure not only a measurement model is developed, but the choice of a predictor (namely academic achievement) is implied as well.

The main advantage of this procedure is that no complicated calculations are needed. However, the disadvantages are also obvious (Applebee, 1971; Reynolds, 1984). One of the problems is defining the cut-off: what is to be considered as an important discrepancy? Choices are arbitrary. Another problem is that the model suggests that the rate of learning is constant during the academic year. But several studies have documented the occurence of growth spurts especially in Grades 1 and 2. Nevertheless, this model is frequently used for sampling purposes as well as in clinical practice.

In the second group of measurement models achievement is predicted and then compared to actual performance. The significance of the difference is tested. Several variants of this model have been developed. We shall mention two of them.

The first is the so-called simple difference model. It is recommended by Reynolds (1984) as a simple alternative to the "two years behind grade level" model. In fact it is a test of the significance of the discrepancy between reading score and IQ, accounting for test reliabilty. Box 2 gives the formula of this model.

BOX 2

Model II   *Simple difference model*

Y_{obs} = z-standardized score on reading test
Y_{exp} = z-standardized IQ

Y_{obs} − Y_{exp} is significant (and classification is warranted) when

$$Y_{obs} - y_{exp} \geq z \cdot \sqrt{(1 - r_{xx}) + (1 - r_{yy})}$$

in which z = 1.65 (tolerant version; p = 0.05, one tailed)
z = 1.96 (stringent version; p = 0.025, one tailed)
r_{xx} = reliability IQ test
r_{yy} = reliability reading test

The z-values in the formula determine the direction and number of standard errors (the term that follows the z-parameter in the formula) that the Simple Difference must exceed, to be regarded as significant.

However, some objections have to be made. Since IQ and reading performance are not perfectly correlated, equating the expected reading score to the z-standardized IQ is inaccurate: it will lead to overrepresentation of high IQ underachievers and underrepresentation of low IQ overachievers (Yule *et al.*, 1974). Another weakness of the model (and the reason why Reynolds advises caution in using it) is that the standard error of the differences becomes quite small when the reliabilities of the tests are high (say 0.90). This will result in a considerable inflation of the frequency of "significant discrepancies".

One method of dealing with the shortcomings of model II is by accounting for the correlation between reading scores and IQ and applying another formula to test the significance of the differences between Y_{obs} and Y_{exp}.

In model III the difference between Y_{obs} and Y_{exp} is corrected for regression. This difference is tested for significance in a way very similar to model II, but accounts for the correlation between IQ and reading score by adapting the formula for the standard error. It will be clear that this standard error will always be smaller than in model II. The residue of Y_{obs} − Y_{exp}, however, will be larger or smaller, depending on the individual IQ and reading score. Box 3 shows the relevant formula.

BOX 3

Model III   *Regression prediction model*

Y_{obs} = z-standardized score on reading test

$Y_{exp} = r_{xy} \cdot X$

$Y_{obs} - Y_{exp}$ is significant (and classification is warranted) when

$$Y_{obs} - Y_{exp} \geqslant z \cdot \sqrt{r_{xy}^2 (1 - r_{xx}) + (1 - r_{yy})}$$

in which X = z-standardized IQ
r_{xy} = correlation between IQ and reading scores
r_{xx} = reliability IQ test
r_{yy} = reliability reading test
z = 1.65 (tolerant version; $p = 0.05$, one tailed)
z = 1.96 (stringent version; $p = 0.025$, one tailed)

A host of variants of this regression prediction model is available. In more sophisticated variants correction for the unreliabilty is provided. We shall not discuss these models here.

To illustrate the impact of the application of these models on the numbers of children classified as dyslexic we reproduce a table from one of our previous studies (Rispens and Van Yperen, 1987). We applied the three models on reading performance of 399 normal first and second graders (206 boys and 193 girls). The mean age of the children was 87.4 months with a mean IQ score (WISC-R full scale) of 96.14 and mean score on a word recognition test (max. score 48) of 42.9. The results are shown in table 1.

It is interesting to note that application of the simple difference model (model II) results in the identification, as could be expected, of a considerably higher number of children. Neglecting regression effects therefore has an impact on the number of children classified as dyslexic. The application of model II cannot be recommended. For that reason we shall not include it in our study.

3.3. *Measuring a Discrepancy: the Impact of Different Predictors, Different Measurement Models, Combined with Single or Double Discrepancy*

The question we want to answer in this section is: Do different predictors, different measurement models combined with a single or a double discrepancy yield different numbers of children classified as hyperlexic?

We applied academic achievement (grade placement) and IQ as predictors, together with the measurement models I and III described in the previous section (the tolerant version). Looking for the effects of a single

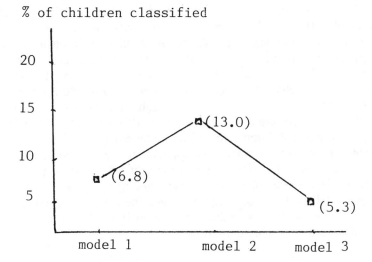

Fig. 1. Impact of three different models on number of children classified as dyslexic.

or a double discrepancy implied a repeated measurement of the difference $Y_{obs} - Y_{exp}$. In model I the first step is to decide whether RA − ERA is more than 20 months (reading performance is the score on a word-recognition test) followed by recording the difference ERA − RA (reading performance is the score on a comprehension test). If again this difference is more than 20 months, the child is classified as hyperlexic. When applying model III (regression prediction model) the double discrepancy implies testing the significance of the difference between Y_{obs}. and Y_{exp}, where Y is the z-standardized score on a word-recognition test; then the procedure is repeated with Y as a z-standardized score on a comprehension test.

Our sample consisted of 32 autistic children, pupils of special schools with special instruction facilities for autistic children. Table 1 shows data about this group and the detailed information is given in the Appendix.

WISC-R (full scale) IQ and two well-known Dutch reading tests were

TABLE 1
Descriptive data (boys, 23; girls, 9; $n = 32$)

	Mean	S.D.	Range
Age (months)	146.50	30.11	87—206
IQ	82.12	13.03	61—109
Reading score (max. 100)	56.15	19.70	20— 89

used. The first is word recognition test (Brus and Voeten, 1972), consisting of a list of 100 words. Children are asked to read as many words as they can during one minute. Test reliabilty is about 0.90 in each of the age groups. The second test is a test for reading comprehension (Verhoeven, 1980). Several versions, according to different levels of word recognition, were used. Test reliability is somewhat lower, around 0.80 for each of the versions. Correlation between word recognition and IQ was estimated at 0.55. The actual correlation could not be used because of the fact that our group consisted of children of low IQ and different ages.

Table 2 contains the results of the application of both models.

Interpretation of this table needs some caution. It may be possible that the models overlap: a child could be classified as hyperlexic by model I as well as model III. Therefore, we rearranged the figures of Table 2 in such a way that the number of children identified by each of the models and those identified by both models are depicted.

TABLE 2
Number of children classified as hyperlexic

Model I		Model III	
Single	Double	Single	Double
1	1	3	3

Table 3 shows clearly the difference between model I and III. The number of children identified by the grade place model is far less than in the case of application of the regression prediction model. This demonstrates the impact of different measurement models on the number of children classified.

This is in accordance with our expectations. Grade placement does not account for those low IQ children reading according to (or above) their mental capacity, but below the average reading performance of their chronological age group. The two children identified by model I as

TABLE 3
Number of children classified as hyperlexic

Model I (but not model III)		Model III only		Both Models	
Single	Double	Single	Double	Single	Double
0	0	2	4	1	1

hyperlexic (and by model III as well) had an IQ of 91 and 98 respectively, whereas the IQs of the six children identified by model III only were considerably lower.

Our first conclusion is therefore that model III should be preferred.

Our second question refers to the difference between single and double discrepancy. Our results are in concurrence with the findings of Snowling and Frith (1986). Defining hyperlexia in terms of a single discrepancy misses an important point. Our data demonstrate that a number of children classified as hyperlexic because of their advanced word-recognition skills, do comprehend the texts they read. Their scores on a test of reading comprehension are in accordance with the expected level. (We used IQ to predict the level of reading comprehension.) In fact those three children had no reading problems: they read according to the expected level. Their performance was in accordance with the average performance of their age group. They were all classified as hyperlexic mainly because of their relatively low IQ: 73, 87 and 89 respectively. Only one girl manifested an impressive discrepancy between word recognition and comprehension: her word-recognition skills were at the level of Grade 6—30 months ahead of the expected level — whereas comprehension was adequate to her age and IQ.

The five children classified as hyperlexic taking a double discrepancy into account do manifest serious reading problems. Their comprehension is far below what could be expected. The discrepancy between word recognition and comprehension is at least — expressed in grade levels — 30 months. In three of the five children it is more than 50 months.

We therefore agree with the Snowling and Frith's suggestion to define hyperlexia in terms of a double discrepancy.

In this study it was not our intention to investigate the other often-mentioned diagnostic criteria, like early onset and the ritualistic quality of the reading. It is interesting to note that in our sample none of these characteristics was observed. In fact only one child did not finish his reading comprehension test because he disliked this type of task.

When a double discrepancy is taken into account, four of our 32 children are classified as hyperlexic. This percentage is much lower than that reported by most of the studies in hyperlexia. This clearly demonstrates the importance of consensus with respect to diagnostic criteria.

4. CONCLUSION

In summary, we conclude that hyperlexia should be defined as a condition sometimes found in developmentally disordered children, characterized by better word-recognition skills than expected whereas reading comprehension is far below the expected level. We suggest measuring this discrepancy by applying the regression prediction model.

It was not our aim to analyze the reading performance of the hyperlexic children. However, our data enabled us to study not only the impact of different measurement procedures on the number of children classified as hyperlexic, but also to get an impression of the reading performance of the group of autistic children as a whole. In fact this study of hyperlexia is part of a more extensive investigation into reading behavior of different groups of disordered children.

Our measurement procedure can be used to identify children with reading problems classified as dyslexic. In this case Y_{obs} is below Y_{exp}. We therefore applied both measurement models in order to investigate the number of children with word recognition below the expected level. In Table 4 the results of application of both models are given.

TABLE 4
Reading problems in autistic children

	Model I (but not III)	Model III only	Both models	n
Hyperlexic	0	6	2	8
Dyslexic	8	2	10	20
No problems				4

It appears that only a few children read according to their expected level. Only four children out of this group of 32 children have a reading performance according to their age and their mental capacity. By far the greater part of the group (20 out of the 32 children included in this sample) has a reading performance below the expected level.

This means that most of the children have to be classified as children with relatively low word-recognition skills. Their comprehension scores are in accordance with their recognition skills.

We conclude that this finding is at least as interesting as the existence of hyperlexia. Hyperlexia is indeed an exception. The most striking fact remains poor reading comprehension.

Studies of perception in autistic children should explain this finding. Research in this field suggests that perception of meaningful information is relatively impaired (Hermelin and O'Connor, 1970; Frith and Baron-Cohen, 1987). Autistic children manifest problems in perceiving stimuli as an organized and structured whole. It seems to be difficult for them to relate the perceptual input to general knowledge and to interpret the stimuli. From this view it should be hard for an autistic child to understand sentences. Lord (1985) points to the relationship between a sentence and a situation. It is this relationship we have to comprehend. We have to relate our general knowledge of the world to sentences. Therefore it is not surprising that autistic children have problems in understanding the content of written or spoken sentences. Hyperlexia should be defined in terms of a double discrepancy.

REFERENCES

Applebee, A. N.: 1971, 'Research in reading retardation: two critical problems', *Journal of Child Psychology and Psychiatry* **12**, 91—113.

Benton, A. L.: 1978, 'Some conclusions about dyslexia', in A. L. Benton and D. Pearl (eds.), *Dyslexia: An Appraisal of Current Knowledge*, Oxford University Press, New York.

Brus, B. T. and Voeten, M. J. M.: 1972, *Een-Minuut Test. Verantwoording en Handleiding*, Berkhout, Nijmegen.

Cain, A. C.: 1969, 'Special "isolated" abilities in severely psychotic young children', *Psychiatry* **32**, 137—150.

Cobrinik, L.: 1974, 'Unusual reading ability in severely disturbed children', *Journal of Autism and Childhood Schizophrenia* **4**, 163—176.

Cobrinik, L.: 1982, 'The performance of hyperlexic children on an "incomplete words" task', *Neuropsychologia* **20**, 569—577.

De Hirsch, K.: 1971, 'Are hyperlexics dyslexics?', *The Journal of Special Education* **5**, 243—246.

Elliott, D. E. and Needleman, R. M.: 1976, 'The syndrome of hyperlexia', *Brain and Language* **3**, 339—349.

Epps, S., Ysseldyke, J. E. and Algozzine, B.: 1983, 'Impact of different definitions on the number of students identified', *Journal of Psychoeducational Assessment* **1**, 341—352.

Frith, U. and Snowling, M.: 1983, 'Reading for meaning and reading for sound in autistic and dyslexic children', *British Journal of Developmental Psychology* **1**, 329—342.

Frith, U. and Baron-Cohen, S.: 1987, 'Perception in autistic children', in D. J. Cohen and A. M. Donnellan (eds.), *Handbook of Autism and Pervasive Developmental Disorders*. Wiley, New York.

Goldberg, T. E. and Rothermel, R. D.: 1984, 'Hyperlexic children reading', *Brain* **107**, 759—785.

Goodman, J.: 1972, 'A case study of an "autistic-savant": mental functioning in the psychotic child with markedly discrepant abilities', *The Journal of Child Psychology and Psychiatry* **13**, 267—278.

Graziani, L. J., Brodsky. K., Mason, J. C. and Zager, R. P.: 1983, 'Variability in IQ scores and prognosis of children with hyperlexia', *The Journal of the American Academy of Child Psychiatry* **22**, 441—443.

Healy, J. M.: 1982, 'The enigma of hyperlexia', *Reading Research Quarterly* **17**, 319—338.

Healy, J. M. and Aram, D. M.: 1986, 'Hyperlexia and dyslexia: a family study', *Annals of Dyslexia* **36**, 226—253.

Healy, J. M., Aram, D. M., Horwitz, S. J. and Kessler, J. W.: 1982, 'A study of hyperlexia', *Brain and Language* **17**, 1—23.

Hermelin, B. and O'Connor, N.: 1970, *Psychological Experiments with Autistic Children*, Pergamon, London.

Huttenlocher, P. R. and Huttenlocher, J.: 1973, 'A study of children with hyperlexia', *Neurology* **23**, 1107—1116.

Lord, C.: 1985, 'Autism and the comprehension of language', in E. Schopler and G. Mesibov (eds.), *Communication Problems in Autism*, Plenum Press, New York.

Mehegan, C. C. and Dreifuss, E.: 1972, 'Hyperlexia. Exceptional reading ability in brain-damaged children', *Neurology* **22**, 1105—1111.

Needleman, R.: 1982, 'A linguistic analysis of hyperlexia', in C. Johnson (ed.), *Proceedings of the Second International Study of Child Language*, University Press of America, Washington, D.C.

Niensted, S. M.: 1968, 'Hyperlexia: an educational disease?', *Exceptional Children* **35**, 162—163.

Reynolds, C. R.: 1984, 'Critical measurement issues in learning disabilities', *Journal of Special Education* **18**, 451—477.

Richman, L. C. and Kitchell, M. M.: 1981, 'Hyperlexia as as variant of developmental language disorder', *Brain and Language* **12**, 203—212.

Rispens, J. and Van Yperen, T. A.: 1987, 'In search of diagnostic criteria', paper presented at the 3rd World Congress of Dyslexia, Crete, Greece.

Scheerer, M., Rothmann, E. and Goldstein, K.: 1945, 'A case of "Idiot Savant": an experimental study of personality organization', *Psychological Monographs* **59**, 1—63.

Siegel, L. S.: 1984, 'A Longitudinal study of a hyperlexic child: hyperlexia as a language disorder', *Neuropsychologia* **22**, 577—585.

Silberberg, N. E. and Silberberg, M. C.: 1967, 'Hyperlexia-specific word recognition skills in young children', *Exceptional Children* **34**, 41—43.

Silberberg, N. E. and Silberberg, M. C.: 1971, 'Hyperlexia: the other end of the continuum', *The Journal of Special Education* **5**, 233—243.

Snowling, M. and Frith, U.: 1986, 'Comprehension in "hyperlexic" readers', *Journal of Experimental Child Psychology* **42**, 392—415.

Verhoeven, L. T. W.: 1980, *Lees en Begrijp*, CITO, Arnhem.

Whitehouse, D. and Harris, J. C.: 1984, 'Hyperlexia in infantile autism', *Journal of Autism and Developmental Disorders* **14**, 281—289.

Willson, V. L. and Reynolds, C. C.: 1984, 'Another look at evaluating aptitude-achievement discrepancies in the diagnosis of learning disabilities', *The Journal of Special Education* **18**, 477—489.

Yule, W., Rutter, M., Berger, M., Thompson, J.: 1974, 'Over- and under-achievement in reading: distribution in the general population', *The British Journal of Educational Psychology* **44**, 1—12.

APPENDIX

Case no.	IQ.	Months of reading instruction	Word recognition	Comprehension
1	107	112	78	40
2	71	111	50	40
3	91	111	38	38
4	68	99	90	40
5	81	88	88	40
6	101	87	41	40
7	73	87	88	40
8	98	41	70	40
9	89	39	26	26
10	87	37	37	37
11	90	15	12	12

Appendix (Continued)

12	61	48	21	21
13	70	50	9	15
14	38	16	16	16
15	69	62	14	16
16	97	38	28	28
17	103	62	40	40
18	91	38	18	18
19	91	38	85	—
20	70	74	18	18
21	89	85	88	70
22	70	49	19	19
23	72	72	29	29
24	91	39	17	17
25	75	134	23	23
26	70	98	20	20
27	74	80	28	28
28	79	109	19	19
29	75	74	80	40
30	109	50	25	25
31	70	62	19	19
32	81	87	39	39

Scores of tests of word recognition and comprehension are converted to grade scores: scores corresponding with the number of months of reading instruction.

PHILIP A. LUELSDORFF AND E. ANN EYLAND

A PSYCHOLINGUISTIC MODEL OF THE
BILINGUAL SPELLER

0. INTRODUCTION

Information processing models of skilled monolingual spelling (e.g., Ellis, 1984: 73; Goodman and Caramazza, 1986: 311) posit two routes to spelling production, one for spellings that are assembled, one for spellings that are addressed. Following Morton (1980), Ellis maintains that the semantic representation of the word being spelled serves as input to a graphemic word-production system where it activates the appropriate unit which releases the correct letter string. Neuropsychological evidence leads Ellis to conclude that the graphemic word-production system stores all familiar spellings, not just those of irregular or unpredictable words, although Günther (1987) warns against drawing inferences from neuro-psychological data to normal models of reading. Moreover, the existence of synonyms, heterographic homophones, and homophonous but hetero-graphic allomorphs, such as the /z/ in plural ⟨boys⟩, possessive singular ⟨boy's⟩, and possessive plural ⟨boys'⟩, suggests that the translation from meaning to spelling must also be mediated by syntax, morphology, and sound.

Assembled spellings are thought to involve either analogies or pho-neme—grapheme correspondences. Following Campbell (1983), Ellis maintains that skilled spellers use analogies to familiar words when assembling unfamiliar spellings. Campbell dictated words and nonwords to normal subjects who tended to spell a nonword like *prein* as ⟨prain⟩ if they had recently spelled the word ⟨brain⟩, but as ⟨prane⟩ if they had recently spelled the word ⟨crane⟩. The application of phoneme—grapheme corre-spondences presupposes the segmentation of the phonemic string into its component syllables and phonemes, and letters must be selected and assembled into candidate spellings. Assembled spellings, like addressed spellings, cannot be effective without prior syntactic, morphological (Luelsdorff, 1988b), and phonological analysis, e.g., distinguishing the contraction ⟨dog's⟩, from the possessive plural ⟨dogs'⟩, from the plural ⟨dogs⟩.

In a recent version of the dual route-to-spelling hypothesis (Goodman and Caramazza, 1986: 311), reproduced in Figure 1, familiar words are spelled by accessing the lexicon, novel words by accessing rules for phonological segmentation and phoneme—grapheme correspondences, and, for both oral and written spelling the same lexical (e.g., graphemic output lexicon), and nonlexical (e.g., phoneme—grapheme correspon-

R. M. Joshi (ed.), Written Language Disorders, 165—190.
© 1991 *Kluwer Academic Publishers. Printed in the Netherlands.*

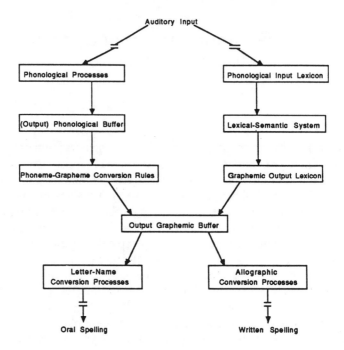

Fig. 1. The monolingual speller.

dences) processes are executed, with differentiation of oral and written spelling (e.g., letter-name vs. allographic conversion processes) occurring only post-graphemically.

The Goodman—Caramazza model of spelling thus consists of lexical, nonlexical, and post-graphemic processing mechanisms. Now, if one imagines this monolingual model of spelling duplicated for the bilingual, in particular for the German learner of English orthography, as depicted in Figure 2, a number of deficits are predicted which in fact occur.

At the level of Phonological Processes, if the English Auditory Input in spelling to dictation were processed as though it were German, and German Phoneme—Grapheme Conversion Rules applied to the phonological representation in the English Output Phonological Buffer, the result would be an English word spelled as though it were German. Ample evidence of this we find in our corpus (cf. Luelsdorff, 1986a) in misspellings such as ⟨Schwan⟩ for ⟨swan⟩, ⟨say⟩ for ⟨they⟩, ⟨sinks⟩ for ⟨thinks⟩, and ⟨fint⟩ for ⟨find⟩, the latter reflecting the negative transfer of German syllable-final obstruent devoicing. On this view, and the one developed in Luelsdorff (1986a), the learning problem resides on the level of English Phonological Processes, not on the level of English Phoneme—Grapheme Conversion Rules, since, for example, if the learner learned to suspend

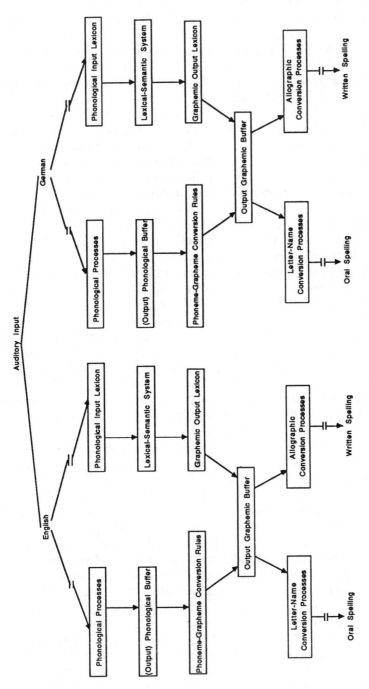

Fig. 2.   The bilingual speller.

German syllable-final obstruent devoicing there would be no problem with assigning the resultant grapheme ⟨d⟩ to the phoneme /d/ in his attempt to spell ⟨find⟩.

On the level of English Phoneme—Grapheme Conversion Rules (PGCs), we find, especially in the first three years of learning, massive use of German PGCs instead of English: ⟨vrom⟩ for ⟨from⟩, ⟨wasch⟩ for ⟨wash⟩, ⟨tschildren⟩ for ⟨children⟩, ⟨jelow⟩ for ⟨yellow⟩, ⟨boots⟩ for ⟨boats⟩, ⟨boght⟩ for ⟨bought⟩, ⟨shauts⟩ for ⟨shouts⟩, etc. Many more examples are available in Luelsdorff (1986a). In such instances there is no reason to think that the deficit is phonological (as in the preceding paragraph), because English and German do not differ phonologically in respect of the misspelled items in question. The deficiency lies rather in the negative transfer of German graphemes to English phonemes similar to German.

For the student of the bilingual speller yet another benefit is to be garnered from the Goodman—Caramazza approach. The component mechanisms of the spelling process may be regarded as modules, since only later mechanisms presuppose earlier and the mechanisms exhibit intricate patterns of interaction and impairment. Besides German Phonological Processes and PGCs interacting with English, in later years of the learning process we find English PGCs standing for one and the same phoneme substituted for one another. Listed under the rubric "bilingual intralinguistic orthographic interference," examples include ⟨Camebridge⟩ for ⟨Cambridge⟩, ⟨jame⟩ for ⟨jam⟩, ⟨sommer⟩ for ⟨summer⟩, ⟨pollover⟩ for ⟨pullover⟩, ⟨braught⟩ for ⟨brought⟩, ⟨enjoied⟩ for ⟨enjoyed⟩, ⟨movey⟩ for ⟨movie⟩, ⟨broaght⟩ for ⟨brought⟩, ⟨wer⟩ for ⟨wear⟩, etc., with additional examples to be found in Luelsdorff (1988a). Just as Goodman—Caramazza (1986: 322) were able to show that the probability of selecting a particular PGC is determined by the relative frequency of its use in the language, and that there is thus structure internal to the level of PGCs, we found that it is in *individual words* that letter-sound correspondences are misspelling-prone (the Word-effect for Spelling Errors) (Luelsdorff, 1986a; Luelsdorff and Eyland, 1989), that the signifiants of two different signs may be substituted for one another if they have the same signifiés (the Identical Signifié Constraint), and that even *ir*regular spelling patterns may be productive — i.e., used to spell words with regular spelling patterns in the norm. This requires abandoning the Dual Route Hypothesis on Spelling and suggests re-examining the Dual Route Hypothesis on Reading.

It has been repeatedly remarked (Henderson and Beers, 1980; Read, 1971; Luelsdorff, 1984, 1986a, 1986b) that beginning monolingual and bilingual spellers employ letter-naming as a spelling strategy. In the case of German learners of English, the letter-naming may be either German or English. German letter-naming includes the articulation of a German letter name, as in ⟨cornfleks⟩ for ⟨cornflakers⟩, and the place of articulation of a German letter name, as in ⟨Jan⟩ for ⟨John⟩. English letter-naming includes the articulation of an English letter name, as in ⟨Her⟩ for ⟨Here⟩, the place of articulation of an English letter name, as in ⟨mess⟩ for ⟨miss⟩, and a sequence of English letter names, as in ⟨could⟩ for ⟨cold⟩. Now, the Goodman—Caramazza model (cf. Figure 1) does envision a letter-name conversion process, but this process is aimed at converting representations in the Output Graphemic Buffer into sequences of letter names, i.e., Oral Spelling. What is needed is a processing mechanism of German Letter-Naming and a processing mechanism of English Letter-Naming aimed at converting representations in the Output Phonological Buffer into sequences of letters whose names properly contain them, i.e., a set of Phoneme—Grapheme Conversion Rules based on letter-naming as a spelling strategy.

Two other, less frequent but nonetheless important categories of error may be accommodated at the level of Phonological Processes in the Goodman—Caramazza model of spelling duplicated for bilinguals. One is the substitution of the English spelling of an English sound which English sound is the nearest neighbor of the English sound to be spelled, referred to in Luelsdorff (1986a: 317) as the Near Neighbor Constraint. An example is the substitution of ⟨ace, ea, ai⟩: /e/, ⟨e⟩: /ɛ/, and ⟨u⟩:/ʌ/ for ⟨a⟩: /æ/, where /æ/ is a phoneme foreign to German. It is suggested that beginning German learners of English classify /æ/ with /e, ɛ, ʌ/ because they are the perceptually most similar sounds to /æ/. This leads to the formulation of an additional constraint on error variables: given any pair of GPCs, where $G_1 = \{L_1, S_1\}$ and $G_2 = \{L_2, S_2\}$, $L_2 \rightarrow L_1$ if S_1 is system-foreign and S_2 is perceptually identified with S_1. Here, we maintain that the near neighbor category of error is located on the level of Phonological Processes because the perceptual identification of S_1 with S_2 is the perceptual identification of sounds.

An example of the second category of error which may be accommodated at the level of Phonological Processes also involves the substitution of the English spelling of an English sound which English sound is the nearest neighbor of the English sound to be spelled. In the first category, however, the sound to be spelled is absent from the native language, in the second it is present, but with a different distribution. Such a case is the substitution of ⟨a, ah⟩: /a/ and ⟨ou⟩: /ɔ/ for ⟨u, o⟩: /ʌ/, where /ʌ/ does not occur in stressed position in German. It is suggested that beginning learners of English classify stressed English /ʌ/ with stressed English /á/ and /ɔ́/ because /á/ and /ɔ́/ are the nearest neighbors to /ʌ/ in the perception of such learners. Such examples lead to the framing of a further constraint on error variables: given any two GPCs, where $G_1 = \{L_1, S_1\}$ and $G_2 = \{L_2, S_2\}$, $L_2 \rightarrow L_1$, if S_1 is common to but differently distributed in the target and native language, and S_2 is perceptually identified with S_1. This constraint on substitution error variables we call the "Close Relative Constraint".

Both the near Neighbor Constraint and the Close Relative Constraint fairly severely constrain the interaction of bilingual orthographies in the case of phonological heteromorphism in the languages involved. since almost all of the near-neighbor type substitutions we have encountered (cf. Luelsdorff and Eyland, 1989, for further exemplification) entail precisely such phonological heteromorphism, it is tempting to claim that the phonological heteromorphism is the cause of the near-neighbor type misspellings. Consider, however, one of several exceptions. The phonemic inventories of both English and German contain /i/ and /ɪ/. In a word dictation to pupils in a German Hauptschule, the main errors on /ɪ/ in ⟨drift⟩ are ⟨e, ie, iCe⟩. ⟨e⟩ for ⟨i⟩ exemplifies place of articulation of an English letter name, ⟨ie⟩ for ⟨i⟩ place of articulation of a German or English letter sound, and ⟨iCe⟩ for ⟨i⟩ apparently the misidentification of unfamiliar ⟨drift⟩ with familiar ⟨drive⟩. Almost all of the errors on /ɪ/ in ⟨skid⟩ appear to be spellings of lax /ɪ/ as though it were tense /i/: ⟨ea, iCe, ie, e⟩. As such they are processed by place of articulation of an English letter(s) sound. The presence of /i, ɪ/ in both English and German and the misspelling of the /ɪ/ in ⟨drift⟩ and ⟨skid⟩ as though the /ɪ/ were /i/ demonstrates that there are near-neighbor misspellings which are not based on phonological heteromorphism, but on place of articulation of an English letter *sound* (*not* name!). With this in hand, we formulate the Adjacency Constraint on error variables: given any pair of GPCs, where $G_1 = \langle L_1, S_1 \rangle$ and $G_2 = \langle L_2, S_2 \rangle$, $L_2 \rightarrow L_1$ if S_1 and S_2 are phonologically adjacent. Since both the Near Neighbor Constraint and the Close Relative Constraint are special cases of the Adjacency Constraint, it appears that the former two may be replaced by the latter. Deeper research in this area, however, may reveal that errors reflecting the Near Neighbor Constraint are more frequent, in which case the constraint should be retained.

There is a further class of spelling errors (cf. Luelsdorff and Eyland, 1989, for some discussion) which cannot be accommodated in terms of the framework of inter- and intralinguistic transfer of PGCs developed above. These include attempts ⟨ham, time, drived [sic]⟩ for targets ⟨hem, tame, drift⟩. Two features seem to characterise such misspellings: (1) they cannot be derived via transfer, either interlinguistic or intralinguistic; (2) unfamiliar targets are being spelled in terms of familiar attempts. The phenomenon is reminiscent of the beginning reading strategy (cf. Marsh, *et al.,* 1980: 342) of using syntactic and semantic context along with partial graphemic cues as the basis for the substitution of a known word for an unknown word, the child often relying on the first letter or the first and last letter to determine the substitution. Since the words in our examples were unfamiliar and occurred in word dictations, neither semantic nor syntactic contexts were available to the speller as aids to spelling. Rather the similarity in phonological shape between the unfamiliar word and the familiar word led to the unfamiliar words being substituted for and spelled like the familiar. This suggests that if a similarity condition is met by representations in the Phonological Processes of the nonlexical route, on the one hand, and representations in the Phonological Input Lexicon of the lexical route, on the other, the resultant spelling will be derived via the Graphemic Output Lexicon. This process, which might be called "Familiarization," occurs within the English portion of the psycholinguistic model of the bilingual speller and is analogous to the processing of false friends, discussed below, in which the similarity of English Phonological processes to representations in the German Phonological Input Lexicon leads to such representations being processed in the German Graphemic Output Lexicon and transferred to the Graphemic Output Lexicon of English.

Goodman and Caramazza (1986: 310) maintain that disruption to the Graphemic Output Buffer results in impaired performance on both oral and written spelling of words and nonwords in the form of letter substitutions, deletions, transpositions, and additions. While letter additions and deletions abound (Luelsdorff, 1986a: 133—200), and they are context sensitive, it is often difficult to tell if the context is purely literal, purely phonological, or a combination of both literal and phonological. What is clear is that the rank orders of the contexts (defined literally) for both addition and omission frequencies are very similar, as shown in Figure 3, indicating that whatever frequency statements attach in the *performance* grammar to addition also attach to deletion. Below, we conclude that there is also no significant difference between misspellings of addition and deletion in the developing *competence* grammars of false friends.

It is also clear that many errors of letter addition and letter omission are products of the orthography/phonology interface. In terms of vowel letters added (Luelsdorff, 1986a: 136) 67% consist in the addition of ⟨e⟩, almost 50% in C __ ≠ position, and almost 50% in C __ V. Closer inspection of the ⟨e⟩-addition errors in C __ ≠ reveals that they are *not*

	Vowel additions	*Vowel omissions*
	C _____ C	C _____ ≠
Frequency	C _____ ≠	C _____ C
	C _____ V	V _____ C
	V _____ C	C _____ V
	V _____ ≠	V _____ ≠
	≠ _____ C	≠ _____ C
	V _____ V	V _____ V
	≠ _____ V	≠ _____ V

Fig. 3. Ranked contexts by frequency of vowel additions and omissions

attributable to regularization to primary vowel-patterns in ⟨—VCe≠⟩, involving as it does augmentation by ⟨-e⟩, as, for example, ⟨righte⟩ for ⟨right⟩ might suggest, but to the *phonetic* spelling of (1) English allophonic aspiration of word-final voiceless noncontinuant obstruents, as in the attempts ⟨pute, leate, lefte⟩ for the targets ⟨put, late, left⟩, (2) the *phonetic* spelling of carefully articulated or spelled nasals and semivowels, as in attempts ⟨ice-creame, theye⟩ for targets ⟨ice-cream, they⟩, and (3) over generalizations of secondary vowel-patterns to primary, as in ⟨newyspe*a*per, le*a*te⟩ for ⟨newsp*a*per, l*a*te⟩. Since category (3) entails a secondary vowel-pattern representation of a single vowel sound (diphthong), this error type is perhaps better regarded as instantiating a substitution rather than an addition. There is thus little doubt that some errors of letter addition are phonetically motivated and that the context of such errors is phonetic or phonological, rather than graphemic. Consequently, the input to the error mechanism of addition cannot be the Phonological Output Buffer, as Goodman and Caramazza propose, but the Phonological Output Buffer containing phonetic and phonological representations. In terms of vowel letters omitted, 83% consist in the omission of ⟨e⟩, 46% in C __ ≠ position, and 43% in C __ V, rendering ⟨e⟩ that vowel which is most favored under both misaddition and misomission and C __ ≠ the most favored environment for that vowel. Closer inspection of the omissions of ⟨e⟩ in C __ ≠ reveals that the majority of these omissions can be explained in terms of English and German letter-naming as a spelling strategy, for example ⟨Her⟩ for ⟨Here⟩ (English letter-naming) and ⟨Hir⟩ (German letter-naming) and the negative transfer of German GPCs, as in ⟨Preis⟩ for ⟨prize⟩ and ⟨prais⟩ for ⟨prize⟩. Here, the engagement of one or another processing strategy, English or German letter-naming, or German PGCs, triggers the error mechanism of substitution which, in turn, triggers the error mechanism of omission.

Like additions and omissions, letter substitutions cannot be stated in terms of letters alone (Luelsdorff, 1986a: 75—132, 265—322), but rather in terms of a letter signifiant X being substitutable for a letter signifiant Y if X and Y have the same or similar signifiés. For example, if ⟨u⟩ spells /U/ in the norm, as in ⟨pullover, full, beautiful⟩, it may be misspelled ⟨o, ou, oo⟩, as in ⟨pollover, foul, biutefool⟩, whereas if ⟨u⟩ spells /Λ/ in the norm, as in ⟨must, summer⟩, it may be misspelled ⟨a, o⟩, as in ⟨mast, sommer⟩. That is, the substitutability of a letter X for a letter Y depends upon the relationship between the phonological value of X and the phonological value of Y. Since substitutability depends upon phonology, errors of substitution cannot be generated from letter strings alone, i.e., they cannot be generated from the Graphemic Output Buffer. Rather they originate from processing strategies engaged on the nonlexical route at the level of phoneme—grapheme correspondences (PGCs).

Errors also originate on the lexical route to spelling which cannot be understood as the result of the operation of Error Mechanisms on graphemic representations in the Graphemic Output Buffer. Such is the case with errors in heterographic homophones. Spelling ⟨one⟩ as ⟨won⟩, ⟨whether⟩ as ⟨weather⟩, or ⟨which⟩ as ⟨witch⟩ does not mean that one has substituted elements of the graphemic shape of the latter for those of the former, but substituted the meaning of the former for the meaning of the latter, i.e., they are errors which must be defined as relations between attempts and targets and their respective Phonological and Lexico-Semantic representations, i.e., information not available in the Graphemic Output Buffer.

We have seen a variety of examples of errors originating on the nonlexical and lexical routes to spelling. Some have involved errors in phonological processes, other phoneme—grapheme correspondences, others semantics. The general conclusion is that errors in spelling cannot be defined in terms of (pairs of) strings of graphemes, i.e., in terms of the Graphemic Output Buffer. Two solutions suggest themselves: (1) error mechanisms (properly constrained) be permitted to apply on each of the levels of processing along the nonlexical, lexical, and postlexical routes — the local solution — or (2) error mechanisms (properly constrained) be permitted to apply only to the Graphemic Output Buffer (GOB), where the representations in the GOB be permitted to either inherit or access all representations on the other levels of their derivational histories — the global solution. In either case, the conception of the GOB as a repository of strings of graphemes must be abandoned.

Locating errors of substitution, addition, omission, and transposition (=displacement) at the level of the Graphemic Output Buffer, in accordance with the global solution above, is appealing to the extent that such errors are errors of performance. This amounts to the claim that processing strategies along the nonlexical and lexical route to spelling are the effective causes of the deviant spelling attempts which exhibit simple and complex relations of S, O, A, and T to their normative targets derived via the lexical route on the level of the Graphemic Output Buffer. Once the discrepancy between the erroneous attempt and the subjectively correct norm has been identified in terms of erroneous S, O, A, and D, the speller-monitor may engage the converse of these error mechanisms (cf. Buszkowski and Luelsdorff, 1986) to effect the required corrections, i.e., error mechanisms and their converse.

Most spelling errors made by beginning German spellers of English, however, are errors of competence, rather than errors of performance (cf. Luelsdorff, 1986a: 231). The error statistics indicate that many errors are made in the categories S, O, and A, but few corrected. Taking the fact of an error's having been monitored as an index of its status as a performance error, most of the beginners' errors made are errors of competence. How do these fit into the psycholinguistic model of the bilingual speller?

The essential fact about such errors is that the individual norm is at variance with the community norm. In terms of the psychogenesis of competence errors, either the individual has been exposed to the community norm, but forgotten all or part of it, or there has been no such exposure and the individual has had to grapple with the spelling either by means of the nonlexical route or analogy. Exposure to the community norm followed by competence errors manifested in uncorrectable performance errors is a familiar learning situation. The short- or long-term memory loss operates on the normative input to produce the non-normative intake and output in terms of the familiar elements and relations of transfer discussed above. In such situations where the input $\neq$ intake, we believe the discrepancy to be *mediated* by the mechanisms of S, O, A, D, triggered by the familiar processing strategies discussed above and elsewhere (Luelsdorff, 1986b). In the case of performance errors, we assume S, O, A, D, to be defined on the level of the Graphemic Output Buffer, since mistaken attempts are being compared with known targets. In the case of competence errors after prior norm-exposure, however, we must specify a normative orthographic (and possibly phonological and lexico-semantic) input, but with an intake *mediated* by processing strategies as in Figure 3.

Figure 4 shows that exposure to the (pronunciation and) spelling of a

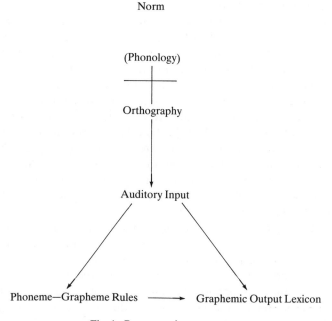

Fig. 4. Preprocessing structure.

particular word may lead to that word being misspelled via the nonlexical (PGC) route in which case the spelling is stored as a competence error in the speller's Graphemic Output Lexicon. The spelled word is processed by strategies which trigger processing mechanisms such as S, O, A, and D.

Thus, the psycholinguistic difference between performance error and competence error is reflected by a formal difference in processing structure. Performance errors (or slips-of-the-pen) are defined in the Graphemic Output Buffer by relations between the norm and norm deviation(s) such as S, O, A, and D. Competence errors after prior norm exposure are defined on the relation between the (non-normative) representation in the Graphemic Output Lexicon and the original, but partially forgotten, normative orthographic exposure.

In our discussion of the psycholinguistic model of the bilingual speller above we have been basically concerned with phoneme—grapheme relations *within* the word, i.e., with orthographic processes within the word without regard for conditioning factors which were lexical, with *sublexical* orthography. There are, however, interlinguistic orthographic processes which are lexical. Such processes we assume under the rubric *lexical orthography* because the speller must dispose of word-level knowledge for the processes in question to operate. In previous work (Luelsdorff, 1986a, 1986b) we divided the data under examination into instances of Cognatization and Decognatization, with each being either Partial or Total, and both falling under the heading of Interlinguistic Transfer. Given two differently spelled cognate words, if the attempt to spell the target more closely resembles the native language spelling than the foreign, then the spelling is an instance of Cognatization, Partial if the L_2—L_1 resemblance is partial (e.g. ⟨preis⟩ for ⟨prize⟩), total if the L_2—L_1 resemblance is partial (e.g. ⟨muβt⟩ for ⟨must⟩). In Decognatization the resemblance between the L_2—L_1 norms decreases in the attempt, as in ⟨Bater⟩ as an attempt to spell ⟨better⟩, where ⟨Bater⟩ bears less of a resemblance than Graman ⟨besser⟩ to English ⟨better⟩. While Cognatization, especially Partial Cognatization, is frequent enough, Total Cognatization and Decognatization are rare.

In the present paper we establish the existence of a lexical route to spelling in German learners of English, in particular that English false friends are spelled under the lexical influence of their German congeners and that this lexical interference is greater in some types of pairs of false friends than in others supporting a new class of interlinguistic grapheme—grapheme correspondences based on interlinguistic interlexical identification. The psycholinguistic spelling models of English and German must therefore be permitted to interact at the lexical level of the Graphemic Output Buffer in the case of lexical items exhibiting a high degree of phonological similarity.

1. THE EXPERIMENT

False friends are sets of lexical items drawn from two or more languages which are similar in sound, spelling, morphology and meaning. For example, the German adjective ⟨allein⟩ and the English adjective ⟨alone⟩ both sound alike and mean 'alone', but German ⟨allein⟩ is spelled with two ⟨ll⟩'s and no final ⟨e⟩, while English ⟨alone⟩ is spelled with one ⟨l⟩ and a final ⟨e⟩. It was reasoned that if such false friends exhibited a higher incidence of spelling errors than nonfalse friend controls, then the relative learning complexity of the target language false friends would be due to their similarity with their native language congeners, and the English spellings in question would be accessed via their German partners. If the incidence of error on different types of false friends significantly differs, then different classes of false friends must be assigned different transfer probabilities. Finally, if the error incidence indicated that some operations, such as addition, needed to generate English false friends from German were more error-prone than others, such as deletion, then it would be necessary to assign such operations a higher rank in the hierarchy of interlinguistic grapheme—grapheme relations.

For example, assume that English medial doubled consonants are significantly more frequently singled in false friends like ⟨gallery⟩ (cf. German ⟨Galerie⟩) than in nonfalse friends and that this false-friend error-proneness was due to target language-native language similarity. Next assume that English medial doubled consonants (⟨gallery⟩) are significantly more frequently singled than word-final doubled consonants like ⟨grass⟩ (cf. German false friend ⟨Gras⟩). If ⟨—CC—⟩, as in ⟨gallery⟩, was inherently orthographically more complex than another type of false friend containing (—CC≠), as in ⟨grass⟩, i.e. that the learning of medial orthographic geminates occurred at a later developmental stage than the learning of final orthographic geminates. Finally, assume that the incidence of error on medial consonant gemination in false friends like ⟨gallery⟩ is higher than on medial consonant singling in false friends like ⟨alone⟩ (cf. German ⟨allein⟩). If this were representative, we would conclude that the operation of letter addition required to convert the single ⟨l⟩ in German ⟨Galerie⟩ to the double ⟨ll⟩ in English ⟨gallery⟩ is inherently more difficult than the operation of letter deletion required to convert the double ⟨ll⟩ in German ⟨allein⟩ to the single ⟨l⟩ in English ⟨alone⟩. Such results would follow from a theory of complexity in which it was stipulated that (1) false friends are more complex than nonfalse friends, (2) medial geminate consonant spellings are more complex than final geminate consonants, (3) letter additions are more complex than letter omissions, and (4) familiar words are less error-prone than unfamiliar.

A word dictation consisting of 74 items (cf. Appendix 1) was presented by the regular classroom teacher to an intact class of 23 pupils in Grade 9 of the German Gymnasium. The items on the test were all real English words, randomized according to a table of random numbers. Unfamiliar real words are marked with an asterisk. The words were divided into six test groups (Appendix 2) and six corresponding control groups (Appendix 3). The test groups were labelled A, A', B, B', C, and C'. Belonging to test group A were those English false friends which end in a final ⟨−e ≠⟩, corresponding to German false friends without a final ⟨−e ≠⟩. Examples include English ⟨culture⟩, corresponding to German ⟨Kultur⟩, and English ⟨medicine⟩, corresponding to German ⟨Medizin⟩. In test group A' were words with no final ⟨−e ≠⟩ in English, corresponding to false friends with a final ⟨−e ≠⟩ in German. For example, English ⟨address⟩ corresponding to German ⟨Adresse⟩. In test group B were words with a final ⟨−CC ≠⟩ in English, corresponding to German false friends with a final ⟨−C ≠⟩. Examples include English ⟨grass⟩ corresponding to German ⟨Gras⟩ and English ⟨staff⟩ corresponding to German ⟨Stab⟩. Belonging to group B' were English words ending in a final ⟨−C ≠⟩, corresponding to German false friends ending in a final ⟨−CC ≠⟩. Examples include English ⟨violet⟩, corresponding to German ⟨Violett⟩, and English ⟨rebel⟩ corresponding to German ⟨Rebell⟩. Group C includes English words in medial ⟨−CC−⟩, corresponding to German words in medial ⟨−C−⟩. Examples are English ⟨gallery⟩, corresponding to German ⟨Galerie⟩, and English ⟨cannon⟩, corresponding to German ⟨Kanone⟩. Finally, group C' consisted of English words in medial ⟨−C−⟩, corresponding to German words in medial ⟨−CC−⟩. Examples here include English ⟨weapon⟩, corresponding to German ⟨Waffen⟩, and English ⟨career⟩ corresponding to German ⟨Karriere⟩. The entire corpus of test words is presented in Appendix 2 and the entire corpus of control words is presented in Appendix 3.

It will be noted that A, B, and C differ from A', B', and C' in one essential respect. The items in the former group, from the point of view of German, all contain letter *additions*. The items in the latter group, from the point of view of German, all contain letter *deletions*. If it can be shown that there is interlexical transfer from German to English — i.e., either that a German lexical item is being inserted into the English lexicon or that a German lexical item in the German lexicon is being accessed while English is being spelled — then it would follow that the English items in A, B, and C are being spelled, when spelled correctly, by means of an orthographic rule of addition, while the English words in A', B', and C', when spelled correctly, are being spelled by means of an orthographic rule of deletion. Looking at the English items independently of German, it is not obvious that either addition or deletion should be involved. English ⟨genitive⟩, for example, appears to have a final ⟨−e ≠⟩ which is either lexical (not rule governed) or spelled by means of a general rule attaching ⟨−e ≠⟩ to words otherwise ending in ⟨v or ⟨u⟩, i.e., not one which results from its addition in relation to its absence from German. ⟨method⟩, to take another example, appears to simply end in a ⟨d⟩, rather than in a ⟨ɸ⟩ resulting from the deletion of ⟨—e ≠⟩ from German.

Some words belonged to more than one of the groups A, B, C, A′, B′, C′. For example, ⟨alone⟩ belongs to group A as it ends in a final ⟨—e ≠⟩ whereas the corresponding German word ⟨allein⟩ does not. As well, ⟨alone⟩ belongs to group C′ because it has a single medial ⟨l⟩ whereas the German word ⟨allein⟩ has a double medial ⟨l⟩. The basis of the experiment, then, was not single words but rather orthographic features. The number of correct spellings per feature was obtained. For the word ⟨alone⟩, all 23 participants used a final ⟨—e ≠⟩, whereas four of the participants used ⟨ll⟩ instead of ⟨l⟩. Hence as a member of group A, the number of correct spellings was 23 whereas as a member of group C′, the number of correct spellings was 19. In all the number of orthographic features was 112.

2. THE RESULTS

The four hypotheses were assessed together by modelling the proportion of correct spellings in terms of nearness to German, orthographic type and word familiarity. These are defined in Table 1. Analysis of variance techniques were used with response variable being arcsin $\{p\}$, where p is the proportion of correct spellings.

TABLE 1

Nearness to German	test: a similar German word exists	
	control: a similar German word does not exist	
Type	—e ≠	Present in one of the words in the English—German
	—CC ≠	word-pair
	—CC—	
Operation	addition: in English—German word-pairs, English has extra letter	
	deletion: in English—German word-pairs, German has extra letter	
Familiarity	English word to be spelled is familiar or unfamiliar	

The first hypothesis is supported ($F(3.5)$, $df(3, 35)$, $p < 0.02$). Words which had a German neighbor (test word) were less likely to be spelled correctly than words without a German neighbor (control words). This is made clear in Table 2 where we compare test with control words for the two sets of words, familiar and unfamiliar, separately.

The second hypothesis that error proneness is related to orthographic type is supported ($F = 6.0$, $df(2, 35)$, $p < 0.006$). In this analysis, only words with a German neighbor were used, i.e., test words. Words with ⟨—e ≠⟩ were less error-prone than words with ⟨—C ≠⟩ which were less error-prone than words with ⟨—C—⟩. The result persisted even when

TABLE 2

	Nearness to German	size	mean	s.d.
familiar	test	25	16.2	5.7
	control	17	19.2	4.3
unfamiliar	test	13	12.0	4.5
	control	57	14.8	7.5

allowance was made for the disparity in the number of familiar and unfamiliar words between the two groups ($F(4.9)$, df $(2, 34)$, $p < 0.01$).

The third hypothesis that orthographic operation is associated with correct spelling is not supported. Again, this hypothesis was assessed using only the test words. Adjustment was made for both word familiarity and orthographic type ($F(0.61)$, $df(3, 31)$, $p < 0.61$).

The fourth hypothesis that familiar words are more likely to be spelled correctly than unfamiliar words is strongly supported as can be seen from Table 2.

3. DISCUSSION

Comparison of the test and control scores indicates that spelling performance is poorer on each of the six categories of false friends than on the matched, nonfalse friend controls, despite the fact that almost all of the controls were unfamiliar words. The sole exception is English final $\langle -CC \neq \rangle$. The control items in question are (56) $\langle$embarra*ss*$\rangle$ and (57) $\langle$succe*ss*$\rangle$, a familiar word was correctly spelled on 19/23 occasions. It is thus possible that if the control corpus had been larger and/or consisted only of familiar words, the performance would have been better on $\langle -CC \neq \rangle$ controls than on the corresponding false-friend test words.

This false-friend inferiority effect requires an explanation. We submit that the *lexical phonological similarity* between the auditory L_2 intake and the stored L_1 false-friend pronunciation is the responsible common denominator, since it is this *lexical phonological similarity* which distinguishes the false friends in the test group from the nonfalse friends in the controls.

This interlinguistic theory of lexical transfer of false friends receives strong support from a consideration of test groups A', B', C, and C'. In test group A' are English items without a final $\langle -e \neq \rangle$ ($\langle$cannon$\varnothing\rangle$) corresponding to German items with a final $\langle -e \neq \rangle$ ($\langle$Kanon*e*$\rangle$). There is nothing in the *phonological* structure of the English items which would motivate a final $\langle -e \neq \rangle$. Consequently, we attribute the frequent English misspelling in final $\langle -e \neq \rangle$ to the association of the English auditory inputs with their German false-friend lexical counterparts. The fact that this interlinguistic interlexical association applies to both familiar (⟨address, control⟩) and unfamiliar (⟨cannon, medal⟩) lexical items with roughly equal frequency indicates that interlinguistic interlexical transfer of orthography is, at this level of learning, quite indifferent to familiarity. The errors in groups B′, C, C′ could be due to the negative transfer of German consonant singling and doubling (but cf. Luelsdorff and Eyland, 1989), but this hypothesis would leave unexplained why the percentages of error on the test words are so much higher than on the controls. This test-control error differential leads us to conclude that false friends are subject to interlinguistic interlexical transfer, rather than the transfer of native language PGCs, in this case German consonant singling and doubling.

The explanation of the type results poses a formidable problem to the theory of orthographic universals (Justeson, 1977; Volkov, 1982). According to Ferguson (1984), implicational universals contain an antecedent term which is more complex, more difficult to learn, and, consequently, more error-prone. In the context of the data above, one relevant universal is Volkov (23), according to which," "If there is a complex unilateral syntagm, then there is a simple unilateral syntagm."

On Volkov (23), orthographic strings containing geminate consonants (complex), which determine the shortness of the pronunciation of the preceding vowel (unilateral syntagm), are more complex and hence should be learned later than single orthographic consonants (simple), which determine the length of the preceding vowel (unilateral syntagm). In point of fact, however, whereas English medial ⟨—CC—⟩s are performed on worse than English medial ⟨—C—⟩s, English final ⟨—CC≠⟩s are performed on better than English final ⟨—C≠⟩s, the latter in contradiction to the prediction made by the orthographic universal Volkov (23). Nor does it remedy the situation to view this result solely in terms of German, for while the corresponding German false friends in final ⟨—C≠⟩s are indeed performed on better than those in final ⟨—CC≠⟩s, German false friends in medial ⟨—C—⟩s are performed on worse than German false friends in medial ⟨—CC—⟩s, the latter also in contradiction to the prediction of orthographic universal Volkov (23). Thus, neither the English nor the German false friends can be said to support the theory of orthographic universals on this point.

Moreover, the data contradict the predictions of universal orthography on a second point. According to Volkov (19) "If there is a progressive syntagm, there is also a regressive syntagm (a regressive syntagm may be found without a progressive, but not vice-versa)."

Accordingly, progressive syntagms should be more complex, more error-prone, and harder to learn than regressive.

Now, most of the data in (A), with a final ⟨—e≠⟩ in English, but no final ⟨—e≠⟩ in German-related false friends, results from the addition of

$\langle -e \neq \rangle$ to otherwise final $\langle -u \neq, -v \neq \rangle$, i.e., the addition of graphotactic $\langle e \rangle$, as pointed out by Venezky (1970). If this is so, then there is a syntagmatic relation between the $\langle u, v \rangle$ and the following $\langle e \rangle$ such that the presence of $\langle e \rangle$ is progressively determined by the preceding $\langle u, v \rangle$. According to Volkov (23), this progressive relation should be more complex, harder to learn, and more error-prone than either consonant singling (B′, C′) or consonant doubling (B, C), but, contrary to the predictions of Volkov (23), the very opposite is true: final $\langle -e \neq \rangle$ is learned first, then consonant singling and doubling in final position, then consonant singling and doubling in medial position. Evidently, the theory of orthographic universals is in need of emendation or revision so that its predictions correspond to the facts. Several aspects seem worth considering. One is that there are cognates in German and English with final $\langle -e \neq \rangle$ in German ($\langle$Adresse, Kanone, Kontrolle, medaille$\rangle$, etc.), with no final $\langle -e \neq \rangle$ or schwa-like sound in English ($\langle$address, cannon, control, medal$\rangle$, etc.). These words appear simple because of the nature of English and the English—German relation. Other items have no $\langle -e \neq \rangle$ in German ($\langle$allein, Literatur, Genitiv$\rangle$, etc.), but have English cognates with silent final $\langle -e \neq \rangle$ ($\langle$alone, literature, genitive$\rangle$, etc.). These items seem easy to learn because the final $\langle -e \neq \rangle$, although silent, is regular in the sense that it appears either after otherwise final $\langle u, v \rangle$, after cognates of German words ending in $\langle -ur, -in \rangle$, or in major secondary spellings $\langle -ore, -one \rangle$. Taken together, it is these relations between English and German which are easier to learn than those found in cognate consonant doubling and singling. In respect of consonant doubling and singling in final and medial positions, the data suggest that final position is a simpler position than medial position, especially for consonant doubling. If these various syntagmatic and positional effects are repeatedly upheld, then it appears that they ought to have a place in orthographic universals if the theory of orthographic universals is to explain the facts of orthography acquisition.

Assuming that the interlinguistic interlexical transfer hypothesis is correct, we further conclude that the English items in Groups A, B, and C are interlexically orthographically processed by *orthographic additions*, while the English items in groups A′, B′, and C′ are interlexically orthographically processed by *orthographic deletions*. In the former case (A, B, C), this implies that the final $\langle -e \neq \rangle$ in words of the type $\langle$genitive, passive$\rangle$ is neither learned by rote nor as a result of the rule that words otherwise ending in $\langle u, v \rangle$ take a final graphotactic $\langle -e \neq \rangle$, but rather by learning that certain German words like $\langle$Genitiv, Magazin$\rangle$ have cognate English words in $\langle -e \neq \rangle$. With the acquisition of fluent English spelling, however, it is likely that this German orthographic base is abandoned in favor of one that is strictly English. Conversely, in the case of groups A′, B′, and C′ the implication is that the spellings of the English items are learned via deletions from the spellings of the German cognates, rather than independently. Thus, English ⟨address⟩ is learned via deletion of the ⟨—e≠⟩ from German ⟨Adresse⟩, English ⟨violet⟩ via the deletion of the ⟨t≠⟩ from German ⟨Violett⟩, and English ⟨alone⟩ via the deletion of the ⟨—l—⟩ from German ⟨allein⟩.

Our previous taxonomy of processing strategies in the incipient bilingual speller (Luelsdorff, 1986b, 1987a) envisages processing strategies that are interlinguistic and intralinguistic. The interlinguistic processing strategies are sublexical and lexical. The sublexical strategies are German letter-naming (Luelsdorff, 1984) and the employment of German PGCs. In the information processing model of the bilingual speller, German letter-naming and German PGCs must be taken to interact with English letter-naming and English PGCs. The lexical processing strategies, in addition to the spelling of items which cannot be sublexically derived, have been termed partial and total cognatization (Luelsdorff, 1986a). In the present paper, we have shown that a subclass of cognates termed "false friends" is significantly more error-prone in the spelling of the German learner of English than otherwise matched items that are not false friends. This led us to conclude that the English auditory input is associated with the German input lexicon where the items in question are associated with German orthographic representations, either resulting in an English/German cognate spelled as though it were German (total cognatization), or spelled part German, part English (partial cognatization), or spelled in English as a result of derivation via addition and deletion from German, i.e., correctly, but for the wrong reasons.

4. CONCLUSION

The above considerations lead us to the psycholinguistic model of the bilingual speller presented in Figure 5.

This bilingual model is similar to monolingual models in that it incorporates nonlexical, lexical, and postlexical processing *routes*. The nonlexical route is for spelling unfamiliar words, the lexical route for spelling familiar words; and the postlexical route for oral or written spelling. Moreover, the bilingual model incorporates the processing *levels* of each of the three routes of the monolingual model.

It was found that the monolingual model had to be enriched by a level of Morphological Processes (MP) along the nonlexical route and Morphological Structure (MS) along the lexical route, because there are words in English which cannot be correctly spelled without reference to their morphological structure. Secondly, we found that the monolingual model had to be enriched by levels and relations permitting the production, detection, and correction of orthographic errors of performance and competence. Processing strategies are responsible for the production of such errors along both the nonlexical and lexical routes to spelling, and

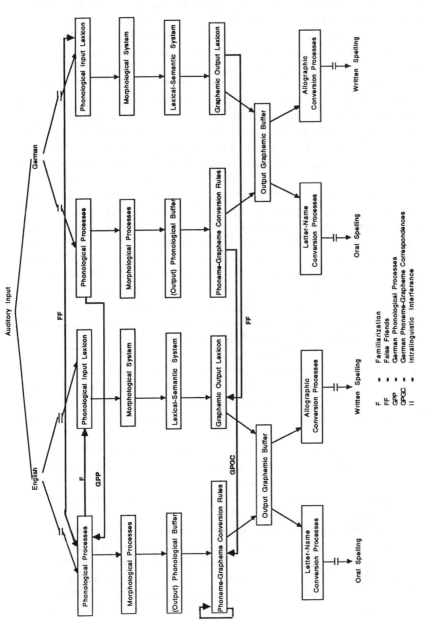

Fig. 5. The beginning bilingual speller.

errors are recognized as such in the Graphemic Output Buffer (GOB) by means of defining the relations of S, O, A, and D there between attempts and targets. In order for this comparison to be effective, it is essential for the graphemic representations in the GOB to be able to access the various types of linguistic information contained on all the levels of the routes from which they are derived, a view which we have referred to as the "global position." Once the relation(s) have been defined and the error(s) thereby detected, the speller is free to engage the converse of the relations in questions in order to effect error correction. On a correct-error perception, error correction reverses the error relations defined on the pair (attempt, target), yielding an attempt which is the same as the target, i.e., A = T. Such an attempt, edited to conform to a target, is then free to either undergo Letter-Name Conversion (LNC) in Oral Spelling (OS) or Allographic Conversion Processes (ACP) in Written Spelling (WS).

A competence error is an A ≠ T, where T is a normative spelling to which, if the competence error is to be psychologically real, one has already been exposed. Attempts to (re)produce previous exposures (targets) are, as in the case of performance errors, subject to error, and these errors are most frequently errors of substitution. We therefore suggest that competnece errors be derived via the *non*lexical route to spelling, then stored in the Graphemic Output Lexicon (GOL) of the lexical route. This theory of competence errors predicts that they (1) do not originate via the lexical route and consequently, (2) do not exhibit any errors which cannot be explained in terms of the processes found on the various levels of the nonlexical route or their combination. The correction of competence errors involves the recognition of a discrepancy between an A in the GOL and a normative T in the intake. The nature and sequencing of the stages involved in the correction of competence errors and their ultimate explanation form the subject matter of developmental orthography.

The bilingual model differs from the monolingual in that it specifies three main sources of interference, hence error, from the native language to the target. Two of these sources, GPP and GPCE, occur on the nonlexical route at the levels of Phonological Processes (PP) and Phoneme—Grapheme Correspondences (PGCs), and the third, FF, occurs via the lexical route at the level of the GOB. It will be noted that all three interference processes are constrained by parallelism in that they relate a given native language level to the corresponding level of the target language. The spelling of false friends was found to be subject to interlinguistic transfer because of their relatively high incidence of error. Some types of false friends were found to transfer more readily than others, but the facility of transfer was not found to be predictable from known orthographic universals. Finally, the error distribution and transferability of false friends suggests a category of grapheme—grapheme correspondences from the native language to the target in which additions appear more complex and subject to later learning than deletions.

The information-processing model of the bilingual speller has, we believe, far-reaching implications for the understanding of the L_2 speech and spelling errors of the bilingual aphasic and dysgraphic. Such investigations have often focused on establishing taxonomies of speech and spelling errors in terms of more-or-less defined categories such as syntagmatic error, paradigmatic error, and errors of anticipation, duplication, metathesis, addition, omission, and substitution, and the quantities of each in normals and the speech impaired. The research objective has been to ascertain whether the differences between normals and non-normals are quantitative or qualitative, and to what extent. Söderpalm Talo (1980), for example, arrives at several quantitative (but not qualitative) differences made by normals and aphasics; the former commit more syntagmatic (over 80%) errors than paradigmatic and phonemic metatheses are common, whereas the latter make more paradigmatic (over 60%) errors than syntagmatic, and phonemic metatheses are rare, indicating a weakened capacity for accurate speech planning and a generalized weakened awareness of errors, i.e., primarily a sequencing difficulty in normals as opposed to primarily a selection difficulty in aphasics.

In the information-processing approach to spelling and reading, however, a distinction is drawn between error mechanisms, such as addition, omission, displacement, and substitution, on one hand, and processing strategies, such as German/English Letter-Naming, German/English PGCs, Cognatization, and Familiarization, which are held to be their cause, i.e. the errors are defined by the model in terms of the causal processing strategies delivered by the model, not in terms of the error mechanisms which, on this view, appear epiphenomenal. In addition to being causal, the advocated approach differentiates the same error mechanism in terms of different processing strategies. Thus, while attempts ⟨bost, her, hir⟩ for targets ⟨post, here, here⟩ are all substitutions, ⟨bost⟩ for ⟨post⟩ derives from Phonological Processing, ⟨her⟩ for ⟨here⟩ from English Letter-Naming, and ⟨hir⟩ for ⟨here⟩ from German Letter-Naming.

In the final analysis, it is of little interest to know that various speech productions are instantiations of error mechanisms, because such derivative facts follow from error causation in the form of processing strategies and the constraints thereon.

It follows from the above that any differences between normal and dysgraphic bilingual spellers be stated in terms of the differences between the normal and the dysgraphic bilingual spelling models. The model given in Figure 4 was developed for normal bilingual spellers at the age of 12—14 with German as their native language and 2—4 years of English. The comparison of this model with that of a matched sample of German dysgraphics might reveal differences along several routes and levels, including relatively excessive transfer of German Phonological Processes, German Phoneme—Grapheme Correspondences, German and English Letter-Naming, relatively underdeveloped Intralinguistic Interference *vis-à-vis* Interlinguistic Interference, excessive Familiarization and over-deployment of the processing strategy of False Friends. In short, if the level of explanatory adequacy in the study of the monolingual and bilingual processing of written language is to be achieved, we submit that a causally orientated, processing strategic model be adopted. We hope to have shown in the above that this target is at least worth the attempt.

REFERENCES

Buszkowski, W. and Luelsdorff, P. A.: 1986, 'A formal approach to error taxonomy', in Jacob L. Mey (ed.), *Language and Discourse: Test and Protest. A Festschrift for Petr Sgall*, John Benjamins, Amsterdam, pp. 217—242.

Campbell, R.: 1983, 'Writing nonwords to dictation', *Brain and Languge* **19**, 153—178.

Ellis, A. W.: 1984, *Reading, Writing, and Dyslexia: A Cognitive Analysis*, Lawrence Erlbaum, London.

Ferguson, C. A.: 1984, 'Repertoire universals, markedness, and second language acquisition', in E. Rutherford (ed.), *Language Universals and Second Language Acquisition*, John Benjamins, Amsterdam, pp. 247—258.

Goodman, R. and Caramazza, A.: 1986, 'Phonologically plausible errors: Implications for a model of the phoneme—grapheme conversion mechanism in the spelling process', in G. Augst (ed.), *New Trends in Graphemics and Orthography*, Walter de Gruyter, Berlin, pp. 300—325.

Günther, H.: 1987, 'Phonological recoding in the reading process', in P. A. Luelsdorff (ed.), *Orthography and Phonology*, John Benjamins, Amsterdam, pp. 151—170.

Henderson, E. H. and Beers, J. W. (eds.): 1980, *Developmental and Cognitive Aspects of Learning to Spell: A Reflection of Word Knowledge*, International Reading Association, Newark, Delaware.

Justeson, J. S.: 1976, 'Universals of language and universals of writing', in A. Juilland *et al.* (eds.), *Linguistic Studies Offered to Joseph Greenberg*, Vol. I: *General Linguistics. Studia linguistica et philologica* 4, ANMA LIBRI, Saratoga, California, pp. 57—94.

Luelsdorff, P. A.: 1984, 'Letter-naming as a spelling strategy', in R. N. Malatesha and H. A. Whitaker (eds.), *Dyslexia: A Global Issue*, Martinus Nijhoff, Dordrecht, pp. 159—166.

Luelsdorff, P. A.: 1986a, *Constraints on Error Variables in Grammar: Bilingual Misspelling Orthographies*, John Benjamins, Amsterdam.

Luelsdorff, P. A.: 1986b, 'Processing strategies in bilingual spellers', *Papers and Studies in Contrastive Linguistics* **XXI**, 129—144.

Luelsdorff, P. A.: 1988a, 'Bilingual intralinguistic orthographic interference', *Papers and Studies in Contrastive Linguistics* **XXIII**, 5—14.

Luelsdorff, P. A.: 1988b, 'Orthographic complexity and orthography acquisition', *Prague Bulletin of Mathematical Linguistics* **50**, Charles University, Prague, 3—34.

Luelsdorff, P. A. and Eyland, E. A.: 1989, 'Psycholinguistic determinants of orthography acquisition', *International Journal of Applied Linguistics* **XXVI/2** (1989), 145—158.

Marsh, G., Friedman, M., Welch, V. and Desberg, P.: 1980, 'The development of strategies in spelling', in U. Frith (ed.), *Cognitive Processes in Spelling*, Academic Press, London, pp. 339—354.

Morton, J.: 1980, 'The logogen model and orthographic structure', in U. Frith (ed.), *Cognitive Processes in Spelling*, Academic Press, New York.

Read, C.: 1971, 'Preschool children's knowledge of English phonology', *Harvard Educational Review* **41**, 1—34.

Söderpalm Talo, E.: 1980, 'Slips of the tongue in normal and pathological speech', in V. A. Fromkin (ed.), *Errors in Linguistic Performance: Slips of the Tongue, Ear, Pen, and Hand*, Academic Press, New York, pp. 81—86.

Volkov, A. A.: 1982, *Grammatologija: Semiotika pis'mennoj reči* [Grammatology: The semiotics of written speech], Izdatel'stvo Moskovskogo Universiteta, Moscow.

APPENDIX 1

False Friends: Words to Dictation

Please read each of the following words to your pupils *three* times. On the first reading, ask your pupils to *listen* carefully to the pronunciation of the word. On the second reading, ask your pupils to *write* the word to dictation. After the dictation is over, read the words a third time, asking your pupils to *correct* any misspellings by writing the spelling they think to be correct over the spelling they think to be wrong. Thank you.

* 1. to assure	26. to arrive	*51. to assemble
* 2. gallery	*27. to assign	*52. account
* 3. accustomed to	*28. coffin	*53. attitude
4. alone	29. passive	54. immediately
5. literature	30. telegram	*55. gramophone
* 6. violet	*31. to surrender	*56. to embarrass
* 7. committee	*32. scissors	57. success
* 8. aggression	*33. to appeal	58. buses
9. opportunity	34. weapon	59. model
*10. to surround	*35. to attract	*60. opponent
*11. to approve	36. control	*61. culture
*12. to attempt	37. enemy	*62. apparent
*13. rebel	38. medicine	*63. abbreviation
14. to apply	*39. medal	*64. staff
15. address	*40. banquet	65. interest
16. accident	*41. exaggerate	66. shadow
*17. to announce	*42. career	*67. to annoy
*18. to appoint	*43. to attend	68. metal
*19. to accompany	*44. attention	69. glass
20. to appear	45. according to	70. method
*21. to assume	*46. to attach	71. before
*22. cannon	*47. to approach	72. superlative
23. genitive	48. platform	73. active
24. magazine	49. grass	*74. to accuse
25. adjective	*50. accent	

Starred items were unfamiliar to the pupils

APPENDIX 2

False Friends: Test Words

A. *English final —e ≠*
   German no final —e ≠

4.	alone	alleinø
5.	literature	Literaturø
23.	genitive	Genitivø
24.	magazine	Magazinø
25.	adjective	Adjectivø
29.	passive	Passivø
38.	medicine	Medizinø
*55.	gramophone	Grammophonø
*61.	culture	Kulturø
71.	before	vorherø
72.	superlative	superlativø
73.	active	aktivø

A'. *English no final —e ≠*
    German final —e ≠

15.	addressø	Adresse
*22.	cannonø	Kanone
36.	controlø	Kontrolle
*39.	medalø	Medaille
65.	interestø	Interesse
70.	methodø	Methode

B. *English final —CC ≠*
   German final —C ≠

49.	grass	Gras
*64.	staff	Stab
69.	glass	Glas

B'. *English final —C ≠*
    German final —CC ≠

* 6.	violet	Violett
*13.	rebel	rebell
30.	appeal	Appell
*40.	banquet	Bankett
59.	model	Modell
68.	metal	Metall

C. *English medial —CC—*
   German medial —C—

* 2.	gallery	Galerie
* 7.	committee	Komitee
15.	address	Adresse
*22.	cannon	Kanone

C'. *English medial —C—*
    German medial —CC—

4.	alone	allein
34.	weapon	Waffen
36.	control	Kontrolle
*42.	career	Karriere
*55.	gramophone	Grammophon
58.	buses	Busse
65.	interest	Interesse

Starred items were unfamiliar to the pupils.

APPENDIX 3

False Friends: Control Words

A. *English final —e ≠*

* 1. assure	*21. assume	*51. assemble
*11. approve	26. arrive	*53. attitude
*17. announce	*41. exaggerate	*74. accuse

A'. *English no final —e ≠*

*10. surround∅	*28. coffin∅	48. platform∅
*12. attempt∅	*31. surrender∅	*52. account∅
16. accident∅	*35. attract∅	*56. embarass∅
*18. appoint∅	*43. attend∅	57. success∅
20. appear∅	*44. attention∅	*60. opponent∅
*27. assign∅	*46. attach∅	*62. apparent∅
*47. approach∅		

B. *English final —CC ≠*

*56. emarrass
57. success

B'. *English final —C ≠*

20. appear
27. assign
*28. coffin
*31. surrender

C. *English medial —CC—*

* 1. assure	*21. assume	*47. approach
* 3. accustomed	26. arrive	*51. assemble
9. opportunity	*27. assign	*52. account
*10. surround	*28. coffin	*53. attitude
*11. approve	*31. surrender	54. immediately
*12. attempt	*32. scissors	*56. embarrass
14. apply	*35. attract	57. success
16. accident	*41. exaggerate	*60. opponent
*17. announce	*43. attend	*62. apparent
*18. appoint	*44. attention	*63. abbreviation
*19. accompany	45. according	*67. annoy
20. appear	*46. attach	*74. accuse

C'. *English medial —C—*

* 1. assure		
26. arrive	37. enemy	
	66. shadow	*74. accuse

Starred items were unfamiliar to the pupils.

APPENDIX 4

The Results

Summary statistics for each of the 6 word categories

Category	Test words			Control words		
	mean	s.d.	*n*	mean	s.d.	*n*
A	17.7	4.5	12	20.1	4.0	9
A′	17.3	5.2	6	20.3	4.9	19
B	16.3	3.2	3	8.5	5.0	2
B′	12.4	4.9	7	23.0	0.0	4
C	7.3	2.3	3	11.1	6.3	35
C′	12.6	6.4	7	21.4	2.5	5

INDEX OF NAMES

SUBJECT INDEX

NEUROPSYCHOLOGY AND COGNITION

The purpose of the Neuropsychology and Cognition series is to bring out volumes that promote understanding in topics relating brain and behavior. It is intended for use by both clinicians and research scientists in the fields of neuropsychology, cognitive psychology, psycholinguistics, speech and hearing, as well as education. Examples of topics to be covered in the series would relate to memory, language acquisition and breakdown, reading, attention, developing and aging brain. By addressing the theoretical, empirical, and applied aspects of brain-behavior relationships, this series will try to present the information in the fields of neuropsychology and cognition in a coherent manner.

Series Editor:

R. Malatesha Joshi, *Oklahoma State University, U.S.A.*

Publications:

1. P.G. Aaron: *Dyslexia and Hyperlexia.* 1989　　　ISBN 1-55608-079-4

2. R. M. Joshi (ed.): *Written Language Disorders.* 1991　ISBN 0-7923-0902-2

3. A. Caramazza: *Issues in Reading, Writing and Speaking.* A Neuropsychological Perspective. 1991　　　　　　　　ISBN 0-7923-0996-0

KLUWER ACADEMIC PUBLISHERS – DORDRECHT / BOSTON / LONDON